NEAR HUMAN

MEDICAL ANTHROPOLOGY: HEALTH, INEQUALITY, AND SOCIAL JUSTICE

Series editor: Lenore Manderson

Books in the Medical Anthropology series are concerned with social patterns of and social responses to ill health, disease, and suffering, and how social exclusion and social justice shape health and healing outcomes. The series is designed to reflect the diversity of contemporary medical anthropological research and writing and will offer scholars a forum to publish work that showcases the theoretical sophistication, methodological soundness, and ethnographic richness of the field.

Books in the series may include studies on the organization and movement of peoples, technologies, and treatments; how inequalities pattern access to these; and how individuals, communities, and states respond to various assaults on well-being, including from illness, disaster, and violence.

For a list of all the titles in the series, please see the last page of the book.

NEAR HUMAN

Border Zones of Species, Life, and Belonging

METTE N. SVENDSEN

RUTGERS UNIVERSITY PRESS

New Brunswick, Camden and Newark, New Jersey, and London

Library of Congress Cataloging-in-Publication Data

Names: Svendsen, Mette N., author.
Title: Near human : border zones of species, life, and belonging /
    Mette N. Svendsen.
Description: New Brunswick, NJ : Rutgers University Press, 2022. |
    Series: Medical anthropology | Includes bibliographical references.
Identifiers: LCCN 2021008397 | ISBN 9781978818217 (paperback) |
    ISBN 9781978818224 (hardcover) | ISBN 9781978818231 (epub) |
    ISBN 9781978818248 (mobi) | ISBN 9781978818255 (pdf)
Subjects: LCSH: Medical anthropology—Denmark. | Animal
    experimentation—Moral and ethical aspects—Denmark. |
    Pork industry and trade—Denmark.
Classification: LCC GN296.5.D4 .S84 2022 | DDC 179/.409489—dc23
LC record available at https://lccn.loc.gov/2021008397

A British Cataloging-in-Publication record for this book is available from the British
Library.

♾ The paper used in this publication meets the requirements of the American National
Standard for Information Sciences—Permanence of Paper for Printed Library
Materials, ANSI Z39.48-1992.

www.rutgersuniversitypress.org

Manufactured in the United States of America

For my parents, Karen and Peter

CONTENTS

ILLUSTRATIONS

FOREWORD

LENORE MANDERSON

Medical Anthropology: Health, Inequality, and Social Justice is concerned with the diversity of contemporary medical anthropological research and writing. The beauty of ethnography is its capacity, through storytelling, to make sense of suffering as a social experience and to set it in context. Central to our focus in this series, therefore, is the way in which social structures, political and economic systems, and ideologies shape the likelihood and impact of infections, injuries, bodily ruptures and disease, chronic conditions and disability, treatment and care, and social repair and death.

Health and illness are social facts: the circumstances of the maintenance and loss of health are always and everywhere shaped by structural, local, and global relations. Social formations and relations, culture, economy, and political organization as much as ecology shape the variance of illness, disability, and disadvantage. The authors of the monographs in this series are concerned centrally with health and illness, healing practices, and access to care, but in the different volumes, the authors highlight the importance of such differences in context as expressed and experienced at individual, household, and wider levels. Health risks, outcomes of social structure and household economy, and health systems factors, as well as national and global politics and economics, all shape people's lives. In their accounts of health, inequality, and social justice, the authors move across social circumstances, health conditions, and geography—and their intersections and interactions—to demonstrate how individuals, communities, and states manage assaults on people's health and well-being.

As medical anthropologists have long illustrated, the relationships between social context and health status are complex. In addressing these questions, the authors in this series showcase the theoretical sophistication, methodological rigor, and empirical richness of the field while expanding a map of illness, social interaction, and institutional life to illustrate the effects of material conditions and social meanings in troubling and surprising ways. The books reflect medical anthropology as a constantly changing field of scholarship, diversely drawing on research in residential and virtual communities, clinics and laboratories, and emergency care and public health settings with service providers, individual healers, and households—as well as with social bodies, human bodies, biologies, and biographies. While medical anthropology once concentrated on systems of healing, particular diseases, and embodied experiences, today the field has expanded to include environmental disaster, war, science, technology, faith, gender-based violence, and forced migration. Curiosity about the body and its vicissitudes remains a pivot of our work, but our concerns are about the location of bodies in social life and about how social structures, temporal imperatives, and shifting exigencies shape life courses. The changes in this dynamic field reflect the fact that the discipline's ethics address these pressing issues of our time.

Globalization adds to the complexity of influences on health outcomes: it both produces and reproduces social and economic relations that institutionalize poverty, unequal conditions of everyday life and work, and environments in which disease prevalence grows or subsides. As Mette Svendsen illustrates in this volume, *Near Human: Border Zones of Species, Life, and Belonging,* globalization sets the patterns of movement and relations of peoples, technologies and knowledge, and programs and treatments. It shapes differences in health experience and outcomes across space, and it informs and amplifies inequalities at individual and country levels. Global forces and local inequalities are compounded and constantly impact individuals' physical and mental health, as well as their households and communities.

At the same time, as the subtitle of this series indicates, we are concerned with questions of social exclusion and inclusion, and social justice and repair, again both globally and in local settings. The books challenge readers to reflect not only on sickness and suffering, and deficit and despair, but also on resistance and restitution—on how people respond to injustices and evade the fault lines that might seem to predetermine life outcomes. The aim is to widen the frame within which we conceptualize embodiment and suffering.

Medical anthropology has increasingly found inspiration in and overlapped with science and technology scholarship—as well as, in recent years, with multispecies ethnographic and other research. In this book, these disparate fields converge. Farming and export industry, animal health, and veterinary science move from backstory to the foreground, with a focus on animals that, as models, stand in for humans in experiments designed to improve human survival and life outcomes. The fate of piglets is tied to that of premature infants, via work on the reproduction of cows and science collaborations across continents.

In this book, the context is, first, that of translational science. The ethnographic settings are two neonatal intensive care units in inner-city Copenhagen. One setting is experimental. Here, sows are delivered preterm of their huge litters by cesarean section and are then put down. Their piglets are placed in incubators for from five days to up to four weeks, to test the value of cow colostrum in preventing infection and death. The second setting, a few kilometers from the first, is an intensive care unit for premature human infants, where clinicians struggle to sustain the fragile lives of tiny neonates as parents struggle to determine their fate in the context of questions of ethics and morality. The cow colostrum formula being tested down the road on piglets seeks to provide an answer to the question of how best to care for such precarious lives. In one setting, piglet infants, near "human" via their role as experimental subjects, are nursed with care and concern by lab technicians, students, and senior scientists. In the other setting, human infants ("near" via their premature birth and their precarity) receive concentrated care and concern from neonatologists and specialist nurses. The goal in caring for the piglets is their short-term survival to study the role of cow colostrum to prevent necrotizing enterocolitis (NEC), a devastating inflammatory bowel disease that is intimately connected to prematurity and is a major cause of deaths in human neonates. The goal in caring for the preterm infants is to prevent NEC and support lung, heart, and gut maturation so that they are able to go home with their parents as soon as possible. The state provides the necessary remedial physical, occupational, and medical support for those children whose premature birth has compromised their health and abilities. So cows feed pigs their colostrum to test whether it might be better than human colostrum to save human lives, and cows, pigs, and humans form a chain of kinship and care.

Our anthropological imagination is captured as we apprehend the tenuous lives of these tiny premature piglets, but as Svendsen shows, other complicated stories elaborate the tasks of substitution and translation that determine their fate. Denmark's iconic dairy industry and pig farms provide the colostrum and the pregnant sows. Danish scientists mobilize international networks of research scientists to set up and conduct studies in China to compare processed cow colostrum with formula to see which best feeds and nourishes preterm Chinese infants. While cow colostrum has already proven successful with Danish neonates on a small scale, the Chinese research provides a large evidence base for the possible global marketing of spray-dried colostrum from Denmark to prevent NEC and ensure that vulnerable infants have fewer infections, good digestion, better cognition, and better life chances. Improved technology has increased the potential survival of ever smaller infants of earlier gestational age, in which context an expanded market for this product in clinical settings would be lucrative. Concurrently, porcine parts regarded as animal waste in Denmark, as well as prime cuts of pork, find new human food markets and consumers in China. Thus, Danish cow colostrum, pork, scientists, and students move to China and back in the work of feeding both populations and "nearly" human and nearly "human" subjects.

Yet there is even more to this extraordinary story of how cows, pigs, and people come together and complement each other in Denmark and China. As Svendsen illustrates, some people are not human enough to be protected by the Danish state because of structural vulnerability and capability. Furthermore, parental equivocation about the life chances of an infant whose health will be compromised influences decisions. This is key in making decisions about the fate of baby Cheung in the introduction, and it is core to extending to refugees and asylum seekers the rights of entry, care, and possible citizenship. In addition, immigrants share their status as outsiders excluded from the Danish state with wild boars: migrating German pigs are kept out of Denmark by fences to protect Danish pigs (which have a high health status) from potential infection with African swine fever virus—which, if identified on Danish territory, could threaten Denmark's pork trade with China. At each point in this extraordinary book, another unexpected connection or complication is revealed.

In *Near Human*, Mette Svendsen brings together some of the most visible, pressing themes and disparate directions of contemporary medical anthropology: interspecies relationships; the transmission of viruses; structural vulnerability; the laboratory and the clinic; ethics and the production of knowledge; and the globalization of science, technology, and food markets. Binding these themes together, this is a story of the negotiation, making, and undoing of borders among humans, as well as between humans and other animals, and the powerful acts of care that sit at the center of new kinds of kinship across species.

NEAR HUMAN

NEAR HUMAN

PROLOGUE

"It is just a pig, why bother?" my friend asks with a hint of annoyance in her voice.[1] We are chatting over a cup of coffee in the fall of 2010, and I have just told her about my ethnographic fieldwork in an animal research facility at the University of Copenhagen, in Denmark, and in the neonatal intensive care unit (NICU) at the university hospital nearby. At the first site, I follow experiments on hypersensitive and highly compromised premature piglets in incubators, experiments that aim to optimize nutrition for infants at risk of the serious gut disease called necrotizing enterocolitis (NEC). At the second site, I follow clinical decision making related to infants on the very fringes of life, some of them born as early as twenty-three weeks gestation. They are the infants whose health the animal experiments seek to improve.

The "just a pig" comment echoes conversations I have had with other friends, my family, and my colleagues in anthropology and public health. When I introduce people to how developments in medical technology are pushing the limits of life across species, everyone immediately understands my interest in clinical decision making and questions about the withdrawal or continuation of treatment for premature infants in neonatology. Just a few introductory sentences about this field immediately provoke outbursts about the urgency of my study, questions about the disability risks of being born prematurely, emphatic responses to the parents' precarious situation, and caring comments about how challenging it must be for me to face the ethical challenges and suffering of families on a daily basis. In contrast to this, when I describe the research piglets—warm and grunting, clad in tiny diapers—people smile or laugh. The fact that I approach the constellation of "just pigs" in incubators with the same set of questions that I use to approach the constellation of infants in incubators somehow appears amusing. What does a social scientist do in an animal facility? In combining these sites, was I signaling a kind of equivalence between humans and pigs? While the research I conduct in the NICU was recognizable to people and had great support, the same research in relation to pigs gave them pause.

In particular, my analytical and methodological strategy of erasing the moral difference between human and animal and treating the animal facility and the

NICU as parallel puzzles most people. This unease points to a moral discontinuity between human and animal that is ingrained in ways of distinguishing between some lives as biological instruments and other lives as worthy in themselves. Particularly in places like Denmark, pigs are relegated to the first category, as a resource for human players. At the same time, my engagement in both the animal facility and the human NICU revealed that a negotiation of life and its worth took place in both sites and that researchers and clinicians make all sorts of connections that disrupt a stable distinction between animal and human. In this book I occupy that space of friction between, on the one hand, practices of thinking and acting according to a dividing moral line between human and animal and, on the other hand, practices in which borders between pigs and humans become unsettled.

At the outset of the project, I shared the conception of "my pigs" as being remote from core areas of public health and medical anthropology concerned with the experience and distribution of illness, treatment, and prevention and the cultural conditions that shape medical practices and institutions within or across societies. However, moving between the animal facility and the human NICU and tracking connections between these sites, I realized that my friend was right in directing my attention to the notion of "just a pig." In this book, the self-evidence of being "just a pig" becomes an impetus to discover how human and pig lives are woven together in social, temporal, spatial, and ethical frameworks. The reproduction of Patricia Piccinini's *Undivided* on the book's cover captures these human-animal entanglements. Although we cannot fully see the animal-like creature behind the boy in the bed, we immediately sense that it is a hybrid creation, and we are drawn to the kinship and intimacy between the two beings. They are not a world apart from each other; instead, they are intimately connected and appear almost as kin. Similarly, the piglets I follow in this book were not immediately visible in clinical care for the children. Yet in substituting for fragile human infants, they became near human and close kin despite—or as part of—the violence that is inseparable from terminating the lives of the piglets at the end of an experiment. When animals become near human in experimental science, how are boundaries between species unsettled and redrawn? How are individuals at the margins of life pulled into—or out of—medical research and clinical care that are meant to save (human) lives? By following acts of substitution, *Near Human* enters the border zones where the very constitution of species, life, and belonging becomes visible.

INTRODUCTION

I am in the operating theater in an animal facility at the University of Copenhagen, a site I refer to as the Newborn Pig Facility.[1] On this December morning in 2009, an anesthetized pregnant sow, washed and shaved, lies on the operating table in the middle of the room. A few days before, the sow had been brought from a farm outside of Copenhagen to the university campus, a transfer that recalibrated her from a production animal to a near human research animal. The sow's tongue hangs loosely from her mouth while two graduate students monitor a drop with anesthesia in her ear to secure her general insensibility. Her saliva drips down on their arms. From the other end of the sow's large body, urine splashes down on the floor. The strong odor of animal body fills the air. The smell of animal does not otherwise dominate the city of Copenhagen. The Newborn Pig Facility is two kilometers from the city center, where flagship stores lie next to trendy cafés, fancy shops sell modish wood furniture, and some of the best restaurants in the country offer Nordic cuisine. In between the city center and the university campus are apartment houses and elegant villas dating back to the early twentieth century. One kilometer from the facility in the other direction is the Copenhagen Business School, housed in ultramodern buildings separated by bike paths and recreational areas. Every year, thousands of students graduate from this prestigious school to enter Danish businesses central to Denmark's open economy, which relies on trade with other countries. Packaged medicaments and agricultural products are among the country's biggest exports, but pigs and other livestock do not appear in the busy bike lanes and streets of Copenhagen. Yet here in the operating theater—within a stone's throw from beautiful old houses containing some of the city's most luxurious apartments—two master's degree students are struggling to sink a knife into the sow's abdomen.

"You need to go all the way through the skin, also through the main muscle, all the way down," the surgeon instructs her students (see figure I.1). As soon as there is access to the uterus, the surgeon takes over and carefully lifts one piglet after another out of the large body. The piglets are miniature, taken out of the womb before term and weighing between 300 and 1,000 grams and still under

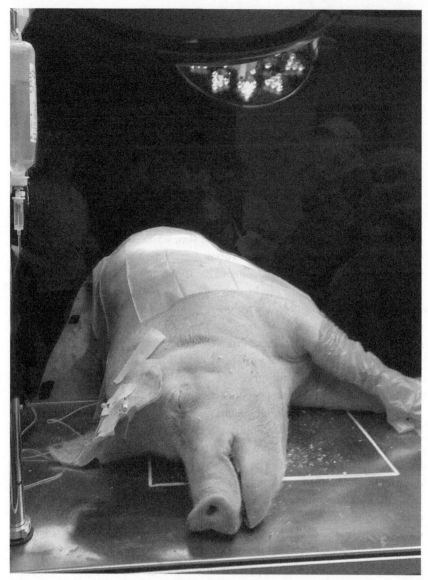

FIGURE I.1. An anesthetized sow, Newborn Pig Facility, 2013. (Credit: Mie Seest Dam.)

the anesthesia administered to the sow. They are slippery. Carefully, the surgeon hands over the piglets to a group of animal technicians, graduate students, and senior researchers, who start massaging the piglets to initiate their respiration and then move them to a separate room. Here the still anesthetized piglets are placed in individual, heated, ventilated, humidified, and oxygenated incubator-like boxes. Later in the day, the sow is killed. The microbes inhabiting her new environment outside the production farm have polluted her to such an extent that she cannot return to the farm. Even if she could, the surgery would make her less efficient "for service"—industry language for her ability to farrow piglets.

After arriving in the incubator room, Christy, an animal technician, is responsible for weighing the piglets and taking their temperature. She gently takes each piglet out of the incubator and carries it the few steps to the scales by placing its stomach on her chest and shoulder as if it were an infant. When a piglet is on the scale, I pencil in its weight on a sheet of paper. Fixing the thermometer in the piglet's anus, Christy moves her palm along the animal's back to provide it with warmth from her hand and sense its condition. A little later, the piglet is fitted with umbilical catheters and oral feeding tubes by some of the postdoctoral researchers. As one of them, Marie, is about to install catheters on the piglet that has just been given the letter L in the Excel spreadsheet listing the whole litter, she notices that it is in a poor state. "It only breathes every second minute," she says. Professor Thomas, one of the most experienced at handling piglets, comes over and watches it.[2] "It is hopeless," he says, referring as much to the piglet's bodily fragility as to the researchers' efforts to turn it into value for science, which will benefit both their careers and infants in the clinic. "Shouldn't we put it down (*aflive den*) right away?" Marie asks. Thomas agrees. Marie quickly prepares an injection and puts the needle right into the piglet's heart to end its already expiring life. A few hours later, upon meeting a colleague who is not part of the team, Thomas jokingly comments, "Today we got twenty-three children." By the end of the week, the piglets have been anesthetized, killed, and turned into biological samples with the goal of increasing knowledge about gut maturation in premature human infants—part of developing new forms of infant nutrition.

Six months later, I am in the neonatal intensive care unit (NICU) at the University Hospital. In Denmark, 6 percent of all live births (four hundred infants annually) are premature births, and prematurely born infants are treated and cared for in NICUs. The University Hospital is only a few kilometers—a ten-minute bike ride—from the Newborn Pig Facility and lies at the intersection of Copenhagen's city center and neighboring Nørrebro, the city's most culturally diverse and densely populated neighborhood. In the part of Nørrebro closest to the city center, lifestyle shops, secondhand shops, and wine bars exist next to each other. In other parts of Nørrebro, blocks of apartments built in the late nineteenth century dominate the urban scene, along with people who are of many ethnicities and ages and speak many languages. Since the 2010s, the cycling path next to immigrants' shops selling vegetables, *shawarma*, and bicycles along Nørrebro's main road has been extended to accommodate three lanes of bikes, yet it continues to be busy. On a sunny day in Nørrebro Parken, the local park, students, marijuana pushers, and middle-class families with children enjoy the same outdoor area and green lawns. The area is also known for gang conflicts. At the time of my fieldwork, a particular Nørrebro neighborhood made up of four sturdy looking redbrick apartment blocks from the 1980s was increasingly seen as a problem by politicians and on the news because its residents had higher than average rates of unemployment and criminal behavior. Although the University Hospital is close to Nørrebro, it serves not only the local area. Its NICU treats the most precarious infants from all of eastern Denmark, the Faroe Islands, and Greenland. Parents come from all levels of society, with middle-class families making up the biggest group—as is the case in Danish society in general.

On this day in 2010, Dr. Karen has just received the message that an infant is soon expected to be born at twenty-five weeks gestation. She knows that infants born before twenty-six weeks gestation have about a 50 percent chance of survival. If they survive, they have 10–15 percent risk of some degree of disability, ranging from cerebral palsy (a form of paralysis in which the nerves controlling muscle movement do not function in a coordinated manner) and visual impairment to compromised cognition and intellectual function. The infant may die during labor, and if it survives, life-threatening complications may arise after weeks or months of intensive care. In Denmark, when a premature infant's biomedical viability and future quality of life is questioned, staff members and parents are confronted with a decision about whether to initiate or continue life-sustaining treatment or employ palliative treatment in anticipation of death. At the time of my fieldwork, for infants born before twenty-six weeks gestation, the hospital guideline listed three options at birth: active treatment, in which case the clinicians do all they can to keep the infant alive, including when it cannot breathe by itself; a wait-and-see approach, in which case clinicians support the infant's breathing if it is able to breathe spontaneously; and palliative care in anticipation of death.

To prepare herself for her conversation with the parents, Dr. Karen finds the medical record of the woman and comments to me, "I need to know if this is the couple's first pregnancy and the sixth IVF [in vitro fertilization] attempt or if it is a couple who already have other children." In life-and-death decision making for infants at this early stage of pregnancy, medical data in combination with family situation and biographies become important points of orientation for moving infants across the border of viability. The "sixth IVF attempt" may shift an understanding of the value of human life and make it imperative to save the infant despite poor prospects. As Dr. Karen quickly reads through the medical record, she learns that this is the couple's first pregnancy, and the infant was conceived naturally. A few minutes later, she and I enter the room of the couple, who are of Asian origin and around thirty years old. The woman is lying on a hospital bed, in visible pain from the contractions, while her partner sits next to her. Dr. Karen talks to the couple about the decision they need to make. Absorbed in pain, the woman does not say much, but listening to Dr. Karen's information about risk factors, the couple realizes that they need to make a decision about whether or not to treat the infant when it arrives. The couple confer together in Mandarin, and the father tells Dr. Karen, "We don't want a child suffering from multiple disabilities." She recommends that they talk the situation through in more detail and says that she will come back in a few hours to continue the conversation and reach a decision with them.

Half an hour later, Dr. Karen enters the noon conference and discusses her case with ten colleagues. The conference is not where the doctors make life-and-death decisions, but where they collectively reflect on the various ethical concerns in individual cases and in that way prepare themselves for conversations with parents. As most parents facing premature birth request full intensive support, the father's categorical statement declining lifesaving care is unusual. When Dr. Karen reports the father's statement to the group, all the doctors around the table find it important that the couple understand that in case of a child with serious disabilities (i.e., brain damage), the doctors are ready to withdraw treatment. "It is important to look the parents in their eyes and tell them that we are not pushing for active treatment if this is against their wishes," Dr. Mads, head of the clinic, says.[3]

During the noon conference, questions are also raised about the couple's attachment to Denmark and how this would shape their child's access to health care and other support the child would likely require. When approaching any parents who are Danish citizens, and thus whose child will automatically become a Danish citizen, clinicians also discuss the three options and are willing to follow a possible parental wish for palliative care. What makes the discussion of the Chinese parents different is that in the noon conference the clinicians discuss the couple's ties to Denmark. Are they residents? Will they have access to public health care? If they have permanent residence, their infant will have free access to health care and social support. If they do not have permanent residence, access to these resources may be difficult. The doctors end the noon conference by agreeing that it is important for Dr. Karen, when she returns to the couple, to ask about their family's social and economic situation.

Later that day when Dr. Karen talks to the parents, they tell her that despite the risks of disabilities, they want the doctors to do all they can to help the infant survive. She also finds out that the parents have been living in Denmark for many years and have full access to public health care and services for their child—which, in the case of brain damage, may include future operations and hospitalizations, physiotherapy, wheelchairs, special footwear, specialized schools, and a lifelong pension if the child cannot support him- or herself. Among the clinicians, the combined commitment from the parents and the Danish welfare state makes the decision making crystal clear: the child is to be saved. During the night, an infant boy who weighs 725 grams is born and is put in a high-frequency oscillation mechanical ventilator. His parents name him Cheung. As I enter Cheung's room the next day, I can barely find his body inside the buzzing machine that sends out a blue light to reduce his risk of brain damage. I am

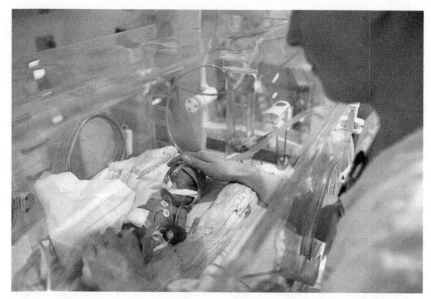

FIGURE I.2. A nurse cares for an extremely premature infant in an incubator, Copenhagen NICU, 2013. Photo by Poul Rasmussen. (Credit: Copenhagen University Hospital.)

reminded of my first conversation with Dr. Mads, in which he described infants born extremely prematurely as "maybe lives" (*måske-liv*). When a child like Cheung is born prematurely, he and his parents stay in the NICU for months waiting for his brain, lungs, and gut to reach the maturity of a child born at the due date (see figure I.2). They live through devastating moments when his situation suddenly deteriorates and raises new questions about continuing treatment. Three months later, most parents are able to bring their baby home.

The beginnings of life in the Newborn Pig Facility and the human NICU are closely related. While pigs are not talked about and do not enter the hospital as living fleshy bodies in the course of Cheung's and other infants' far too early births, laboratory animals en masse populate neonatology. Right after birth, Cheung is provided with the lung maturing milky substance called Curosurf. This lifesaving treatment was developed from populations of pigs whose lungs constitute the crucial ingredient in Curosurf, as well as from populations of newborn lambs (Ikegami, Jobe, and Glatz 1981) and rabbits (Robertson et al. 1990) on which the lung maturing therapy was tested. Another research field in which pigs have paved the way for infant health is hypothermia. Experiments with piglets (and later other animals) in the 1990s laid the ground for what is now an evidence-based clinical treatment of cooling infants who have suffered from a deficient supply of oxygen after birth, thereby reducing the risk of neurological damage (Edwards et al. 2010). A third technical-instrumental connection between pigs and the NICU is the anticoagulant liquid heparin, which is extracted from pig intestines. In the NICU, neonates like Cheung may be given heparin if the doctors need to place a catheter into a large vein—for example, for medication, blood transfusion, or parenteral nutrition.

When I ask one of the doctors about the information available on these medicaments in the hospital's online catalogue, he explains to me that heparin is labeled as "porcine" and Curosurf as "phospholipid fraction from pig lung," but this information does not reach the parents. In the NICU, the pigs involved in Curosurf and heparin lead an invisible life. During my time in the clinic, Muslim, Jewish, and vegan parents, who might be uneasy about the presence of nonhuman species in the body, were not informed of the animal origin of these substances. To the doctors, this invisibilization was not seen as a deliberate act of hiding. They simply did not consider the animal origin important in the context of a stressful birth. Yet, as I suggest in chapter 1, at the same time as keeping the boundary between species is a way of caring for the parents, for me it also provided a way to understand how the human is performed and imagined when life is at the margins.

Although Curosurf, cooling procedures, and heparin represent breakthroughs in neonatology, these treatments' entanglement with animal populations does not stand alone. For centuries, animals have been used as research tools with the aim of facilitating health for humans. The kinship between pig and human that Thomas invoked with his lighthearted comment about the team's "twenty-three children" echoes nineteenth-century evolutionary theory, which established that all living beings are related through common ancestors. As one of the graduate students in the Newborn Pig Facility tells me, "first, we were guts, and from the activities of guts we developed other organs such as arms, legs, brains. Despite thousands of years of evolutionary development, the gut of the pig and the gut of the human are still remarkably similar." His comment articulates a mammalian "we" from which the human "we" develops. In pointing out this evolutionary heritage, he recenters the development of human cognition and morality from being based in the brain to having its origin in the gut. Gut activities connected the first beings to the world and propelled the development of the human. The student's comment resonates with the research in the Newborn Pig Facility, based as it is on the anatomical and physiological affinity between the human gut and the pig gut. This evolutionary relatedness has formed the foundation for proliferating knowledge about physiological and biogenetic proximities between humans and animals. Seeing the animal body as a valid representative of the human body, with comparable functioning of organs and cells, has led to the development of experimental organisms like the piglets. In contemporary biomedical science, the pig is increasingly becoming a model organism that acts as a substitute for humans. Consequently, care for infants in the NICU extends into animal facilities in which the life, suffering, and death of laboratory animals are deeply implicated in creating healthy lives for humans.

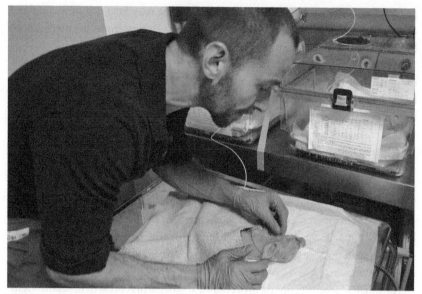

FIGURE I.3. A researcher cares for a premature piglet, Newborn Pig Facility, 2013. Photo by Mie Seest Dam. (Credit: Mie Seest Dam.)

SUBSTITUTION

One morning in 2013 Peter, a postdoctoral researcher, and Anna, a master's degree student, enter the Newborn Pig Facility to carry out the routine feeding of and attending to a litter of piglets born two weeks earlier.[4] The very immature piglets are hypersensitive and compromised beings in need of constant care (see figure I.3). Peter and Anna notice that a particular piglet, referred to by the letter R, is limp and has lost weight. This is critical. To provide good data, piglet R needs to stay alive until its scheduled killing eight days later, and the researchers want to do all they can to achieve this and minimize the animal's suffering. To help Peter understand the piglet's situation, Anna twists her face to reproduce the odd sounds that piglet R was making the day before. "Were these 'sounds of pain' or 'what-is-happening-sounds'?," Peter asks her and then seriously tries to make the sounds himself. In mimicking the piglet's sounds of possible surprise and possible pain and distorting their faces to figure out its situation, Peter and Anna step into the position of the animal and try to figure out how to keep the pig alive with minimal pain so that it can reach a certain future as a research sample a week later. Between what may at first seem like contradictory acts of caring and killing, Peter and Anna attend to the piglets as if they were human infants. Much like caregivers in human NICUs, who take into account the future situation that awaits the infant and family members, the researchers seek not only to provide life-sustaining care. They also work continuously to actualize a future in which the piglet can contribute to science and society. In these critical moments, how do caregivers decide which piglets, or which human infants, qualify for life? And what is at stake for the human actors in these practices of substitution?

In this book, substitution practices crack open the complex ethical field in which life is constituted and precarious beings' attachment to societal collectives is configured and negotiated. Substitution contains a sociomaterial practice of replacement, as when piglets are taken out of the womb of the sow and installed in the laboratory to model human biology. And substitution contains an affective and moral component, as when Peter and Anna twist their faces and place themselves in the position of the individual pig to evaluate its suffering. In this way, substitution brings together two notions of "near" in *Near Human*: the circumstance of being comparable and alike (when piglets are modeled to be almost humans) and the experience of being intimate and close (when Peter and Anna step into the position of another being). Put differently, substitution weaves together the sociomaterial replacement of one being (or part of it) with another with the affective and intimate practice of submitting oneself to another's life, compensating for its inabilities, imagining its futures, and—through this physical and emotional proximity—taking responsibility for that life.[5]

The claim of this book is that substitution practices unsettle and settle boundaries between humans and nonhumans, life and death, and belonging and not belonging. When laboratory practices move piglets into the category of the human, boundaries between species are unsettled and interspecies kinship is forged, yet species boundaries are settled again in bringing scientific knowledge and substances to the clinic. When practitioners in the animal facility and the NICU substitute for piglets and infants, they act as their proxies and take a stance on their lives—thus stepping into the borderland between life and death and drawing the boundaries between them. In these situations, practitioners let piglets and infants not only in and out of life but also in and out of society, thus unsettling and settling who and what belongs in the nation of Denmark. Practices of substitution expose processes of including and excluding different kinds of pigs and different kinds of humans, and such inclusions and exclusions come to define the nation of Denmark and the role of the state in its construction.

"Substitution" means replacement (the word comes from *sub*, meaning "under," and *statuere*, meaning "to set up"). In the Western world, it implies a notion of an original and its inferior. The concept is closely related to Western notions of uniqueness and authenticity and the conceptual distinction between (original) person and (reproducible) thing (Franklin 2007; Hogle 2022).[6] It is precisely because research animals, like piglet R, are not humans yet are close enough to stand in for them that they are enrolled in experimental procedures and become "substitutive research subjects" (C. Thompson 2013, 22) representing "original" humans like Cheung. One of the first definitions of the concept of substitution in the *Oxford English Dictionary* is "the action or act of putting one person or thing in place of another; the fact of being put in another's place" (Substitution [March 2020]). My use of substitution is drawn from these aspects of the meaning of the word. I investigate the sociomaterial practices of putting one being—or part of it—in the place of someone or something else, as when piglets replace infants and medical technology replaces parts of a human infant's body. And I consider how these practices of replacing often involve the affective and intimate experience associated with being put in another's place. I use a palette of related terms—proxy, replacement, stand in, extension—to delineate and unfold how substitution operates in different situations. I make no attempt to understand the pigs' experience of standing in for very sick infants, but I engage the experiences of the human caregivers who mobilize their own senses, knowledge, imagination, and technology to substitute for another being.

In anthropology, substitution is closely linked to the literature on sacrifice. In animal sacrifice, the sacrificial acts consecrate the animal as symbolically close to the original other and thereby move the violence from the original to the substitutes (Hubert and Mauss 1968; Smith and Doniger 1989; Willerslev 2009; Bloch 1992; Girard 1977; Govindrajan 2018). In social science studies of experimental animal research, the sacrifice trope has been employed to describe the termination of laboratory animals for a higher purpose.[7] My concept of substitution is inspired by the sacrifice literature, yet it avoids seeing the human as the default original. Rather, I am interested in exploring the processes of constituting someone or something as original or as substitute and in understanding the slippage between substitute and original. When Christy, the animal technician, gently touches each piglet to keep it warm and sense its state of being, this physical and emotional proximity is crucial to turning the piglet into a substitutive research subject. This aspect of "making [one's] body available" (Lien 2015, 16) is even more pronounced in the situation of Peter and Anna, when they submit themselves to piglet R. Here, the piglet in a sense becomes the original, the authentic sentient being that is mirrored by the humans. Through Anna and Peter's "mimetic performance" (Willerslev 2007, 1) as part of turning piglet R into a good substitute, the human actors come to act as a proxy or substitute for R by literally bearing it under their skin. Such intimacy and affection is echoed in the expanding field of multispecies research that has highlighted dynamic relationships between humans and nonhuman animals in a variety of settings (Candea 2010; Despret 2008; Friese 2013a, 2013b, 2019; Govindrajan 2018; Haraway 2008, 2016; Kohn 2007; Sharp 2019; Willerslev 2007). In particular, with her concept of cosuffering (2008), Donna Haraway has pointed to embodied dimensions of staying in solidarity with and proximity to animals who are in instrumental relations, for example when animals are treated as research tools and undergo suffering. Also, in the context of sacrifice, Radhika Govindrajan (2015) has shown that the consecration of the animal that turns it into a human substitute during the sacrificial process is not only a question of semiotic identification of animal with human but also a practice of intimacy, affection, and interspecies kinship.

As I have already hinted, substitution was present not only in the Newborn Pig Facility, but also in the human NICU. Dr. Karen's patient, the infant Cheung, cannot breathe on his own when he is born. When he is rushed into intensive care, artificial respiration substitutes for his immature organs, and when his situation deteriorates during the night, the head of the clinic, Dr. Mads, comes in to assist in stabilizing his condition—which we may also see as an act of substitution in which sociomaterial replacement interweaves with difficult questions about how far to continue. Even before the infant's birth, the discussion in the noon conference takes us into the moral complexity related to substituting for him. Here, the clinicians not only draw on all their medical knowledge, they also try to step into the position of the parents to seek an answer to the question of how best to care for the patient, a category that in this setting includes both infant and parents. Caregivers in both the Newborn Pig Facility and the human NICU not only reach out and touch "fleshy, fragile, and mortal bodies" (Mol 2008, 31), as may be the case in all forms of care. They also act as substitutes for these neonate bodies, authenticating or eroding their life and belonging in society.

In the last part of this book, I scrutinize the moral stances that come to the fore when policies regulating who and what belongs in Denmark conceptualize particular people, animals, and things as substitutes for people, animals, and things seen as originally Danish. By treating substitutability as a framework for analyzing ideas of replacement and moral practices of bearing responsibility for an other's life, I uncover how in Denmark—across animal facility, human clinic, and migration policies—substitution practices erase a clear distinction between instrumental worth and intrinsic worth. It is because piglets, infants, and migrants hold the potential of entering into reciprocal use relations that they may be allowed into Denmark and become members of the collectivity and gain societal support.

LIMINAL LIVES

Piglets in the animal facility and infants in the human NICU are what Susan Squier calls "liminal lives" (2004). "Liminal" means being at the threshold: in this case, no longer one entity, yet not quite another (Turner 1969). The ambiguity of research piglets and premature infants exposes dominant cultural values about the human and makes it possible to reflect upon and question them. Although anthropology has challenged unitary theories of the human, a central question in anthropology has always been what it means to be human. This question emphasizes the discipline's subject of the meaning-making human (with a capacity for creating culture and exercising moral virtues) in contrast to animals (which belong to natural science). Yet the liminal lives of premature piglets and infants are unmoored from the meaning-making being whom we instantly recognize as human. In her study of life scientists working with chimera-making technologies, Amy Hinterberger shows that the humanization of nonhuman biology "brings into question the relationship between the plasticity of biology and the human person" and that the category of human has become fugitive and cannot be taken for granted (2018, 454).[8] Whereas Hinterberger exposes negotiations of the human in the life sciences, Tobias Rees (2018) asks us to find escapes from and look for openings out of anthropology's humanist framework and rethink the discipline's domain and tools. My approach to substitution practices takes inspiration from Hinterberger's insights and borrows from Rees's proposal. Substitution practices introduce a conceptual shift from "what it means" to be human to "what it takes" to become a certain form of life. This is so because practices of substitution provide insights into the sociomaterial and the affective-moral components of constituting life.

In Judith Butler's books on precarious life (2006) and frames of war (2016), she asks how life gains value. Although her books are about U.S. war interventions after 9/11, her discussions of the frames through which we come to apprehend a life are relevant far beyond her case of the American war on terror. She argues that "there is no life and no death without a relation to some frame" (2016, 7). In suggesting an analytical shift from "what it means" to "what it takes," I wish to draw ethnographic attention to what Butler refers to as "frames": the conditions shaping a life's emergence and value. By adding animals, vulnerable infants, and migrants and refugees to this discussion, I bring her arguments into a new terrain to trace how species, life, and belonging are simultaneously crafted and eroded. Substitution practices, I show, provide a way to understand how liminal lives are configured, valued, and governed, as well as how belonging in a societal collectivity (for both pigs and humans) is drawn and defined. The starting point is that no life inherently has species, value, and belonging. Every life is born precarious and in the hands of the other (Butler 2016, 14), and thus studying how it is substituted for becomes an avenue to excavate life's conditionality and configuration. In this approach, the human is not an ontological entity but "a differential norm . . . that may be allocated and retracted, aggrandized, personified, degraded and disavowed, elevated and affirmed" (Butler 2016, 76). Treating the human as "differential norm" rather than as a self-evident starting point for the human sciences turns the human into questions: How does life gain value and qualify as human? How does life leave the norm of the human?

To investigate these valuation processes, while avoiding the paradoxes of infants who efface the human as otherwise known and piglets that are valued as human yet have the morphology of pigs, I use the concepts of biological and biographical life ("logical" is from the Greek term for "the study of," while "graphical" is from the Greek term for "the writing or narrative of"; Svendsen 2011 and 2015). "Biological life" refers to a configuration in which life appears as biological processes divested from social and moral relations, whereas "biographical life" refers to a configuration in which life appears as a qualified life that is part of social and moral relations; has a past, present, and future; calls for a different respect; and thus can be grieved.[9] Biographical life falls within the recognizable norm of the human. In the case in which Thomas and Marie turn the newly arrived piglets into models of humans and stop to discuss piglet L, piglet L appears as a biological life that the researchers are not yet invested in and that does not have a point of view or biography. In Butler's vocabulary, piglet L is a nongrievable life close to being "socially dead" (2016, 42). In contrast, in the interaction between Peter and Anna and piglet R, the piglet turns into someone—the original that is not simply a biological life but that also inhabits a biographical living, and thus is worth defending and valuing, as well as grieving if lost. Similarly, Dr. Karen's speed-reading of the medical record to understand the parents' reproductive history adds a biography to the infant about to be born.

Importantly, I do not see biological life as the ontological ground on which qualified biographical lives can be established, as the classic Western philosophy has it. Such a view would imply separating the biological from the social and political (Fassin 2018, 66; Franklin 2007, 6; Marsland and Prince 2012, 462; Ticktin 2011, 14). As an analytical approach, substitution avoids this separation since it helps expose what it takes to become biology and biography. Here, I follow Didier Fassin in his ambition to track "the complex intersections and permanent reconfigurations of the two" (2018, 66). Thus, I use the concepts of biological and biographical life to render visible the forms of life that come into being in substitution practices. I explore how human and pig neonates slip between those forms, how the two sometimes exist in tension, and how in other situations a continuum exists between them so that any being may come to contain amounts of both.

In unraveling substitution practices as an intertwining of replacing and stepping into the place of another, I take inspiration from and combine two perspectives that are not usually put in dialogue: multispecies ethnography and the anthropology of morality. These two analytical approaches are closely linked to the two intertwined dimensions of substitution I take up: the sociomaterial component and the affective-moral component. In the following sections, I flesh out my contribution to both perspectives.

MULTISPECIES ETHNOGRAPHY

A growing body of anthropological scholarship on human-animal or -plant associations through time and across landscapes has ethnographically followed pigs, sheep, dogs, microbes, tea leaves, salmon, and mushrooms, among other material, across various sites (Blanchette 2020; Franklin 2007; Haraway 2008; Helmreich 2009; Ives 2017; Lien 2015; Tsing 2015). Through these movements, scholars have exposed the inseparability of humans and other life-forms and have highlighted the interaction between ecological relations and political economies, global inequalities, imperial encounters, and the building of nations.[10] In parallel with this literature, sociologists and historians of science have explored how the development and circulation of animal models is integral to building epistemic infrastructures (Ankeny and Leonelli 2016; Brosnan and Michael 2014; Davies 2012; Friese and Clarke 2012; Friese 2013a; Leonelli and Ankeny 2012; Lewis, Hughes, and Atkinson 2014) and how interspecies relations in knowledge production shape medical knowledge and identity (Kirk 2016b; Kirk and Ramsden 2018; Nelson 2018; Rader 2004). In particular, a proliferating literature on care practices in animal laboratories has explored the entangled subjectivities of human and animal in the making of science (Dam and Svendsen 2018; Davies et al. 2018; Despret 2008; Druglitrø 2018; Friese 2013b, 2019; Friese and Latimer 2019; Haraway 2008; Sharp 2019). Central to all these literatures is an inspiration from science and technology studies, which emphasizes the distributed character of agency and explore how actors (either human or nonhuman) are part of larger "actor networks" that "configure," "enact," or "script" them in specific ways.[11]

Near Human extends these studies' focus on the inseparability of humans and other life-forms to bring into view how life and its value are constituted. Despite a strong interest in coconstitution, multispecies ethnography has not engaged to a large extent the practices through which different life-forms gain value. I address this shortcoming by investigating how the constitution and character of human-animal relationships imply valuations. My method is to juxtapose practices and policies related to various liminal lives. Juxtaposition has affinities with comparison. Yet where comparison in anthropology has moved across geographical distances to comprehensively map differences and similarities, the aim of juxtaposition is to trouble categories and framings (Coopmans and McNamara 2020; Friese and Latimer 2019) that are so evident that we easily forget that "it could be otherwise" (Woolgar and Lezaun 2013, 323). By juxtaposing ethnographies from different sites, I establish "parasitic encounters" (Kirksey and Helmreich 2010, 558), in which practices around one liminal life (e.g., that of a research piglet) become a prism for exploring practices around another liminal life (e.g., that of a human infant).[12] These parasitic encounters are used to expose the edges of a particular constitution and uncover what it takes to become a certain form of life and be valued in specific ways.

Piglet L and infant Cheung are about the same size and equally precarious and fully dependent on others to survive, yet they are treated very differently. Whereas piglet L is placed in relationship to the particular experiment within the bounded space of the scientific institution and the one-week time frame of the study, Dr. Karen places Cheung in social relationships to his parents and their reproductive history and future belonging in Denmark. This may seem like common sense, but in juxtaposing the two cases, we come to see that before the doctors are certain of the commitments from the parents and the welfare state— that is, in the absence of kinship, home, and an open-ended future supported by welfare state health care—Cheung's life has strong similarities to the biological life of piglet L. At this stage, his life appears as a gradual move toward death. As soon as his attachment to parents and society is confirmed, the situation changes, and he is constituted as a biographical life by virtue of being placed in kinship and a home and imbued with an open-ended future in Denmark.

In juxtaposing substitution practices in the animal facility and those in the human clinic, my aim is not to claim that we should include all lives in the category of the biographical life, but to expose the dynamics involved in constituting some lives as biographical and grievable and others as biological and nongrievable. Where a common anthropological approach would thicken the analysis of Cheung and other infants by providing an ethnography of the lifeworld of his parents and doctors, my methodology of juxtaposition creates thick descriptions by interlacing different, yet interconnected, liminal lives in Denmark. In this book, ethnography from both clinic and lab plays a crucial role, yet it is not brought in to understand the lifeworlds of parents of precarious infants or the lifeworlds of practitioners taking care of precarious infants and piglets. Rather, the ethnography offers an account of the experiences and mechanisms of valuating life and making different kinds of pigs and different kinds of humans belong in Denmark.

THE ANTHROPOLOGY OF MORALITY

Unraveling how life-forms are constituted and valuated brings me into the terrain of morality. When I followed practices in the Newborn Pig Facility and the NICU, it was not possible to escape from moral questions. Substituting for highly compromised premature infants and piglets raises urgent moral and existential questions about the worth of life. When Peter and Anna attend to piglet R, they act in accordance with legislation and guidelines that allow piglets to undergo painful procedures as part of the pursuit of remedies to improve future human health, but knowledge of these guidelines does not provide a clear answer to what to do with the limp piglet R. Should it be put down right away— like piglet L, which was expelled from the experiment right after its enrollment? In the case of piglet R, the researchers have already invested many hours in caring for it and keeping it alive, and through this work they have turned it into a model of human infant biology. How can they make sure that the piglet stays alive yet does not suffer too much? How can they make sure that it provides good data, which involves making it suffer? When Dr. Karen enters the room with the pregnant woman and her partner, she is embodying the value put on infant life in the Danish health care system by seeing the neonate enter this world as an infant and not a fetus to be aborted. Dr. Karen knows her guidelines, but they do not answer or make superfluous all the moral questions that are part of the very material practices of receiving a premature infant. As they consider whether to provide active treatment, Dr. Karen and her colleagues ask: What kind of life will this child have if it survives? What are the situation and wishes of the parents? Do they want the child even if it survives with serious disabilities?

In contrast to most multispecies work, the fields of animal ethics and biomedical ethics have addressed the difficult questions of the moral status of precarious beings. In particular, the rapidly growing field of animal ethics is concerned with the human use of animals, analyzing the principles that inform different forms of use, and determining what moral norms should govern human interactions with other species (see, e.g., Singer 1975; Regan 1983). As a field, animal ethics is both descriptive and prescriptive. Through my years of research for this book, animal ethics has been a source of inspiration in my search to understand different moral positions as they inform guidelines of animal experimentation and are expressed by the various practitioners in my field sites. Yet where animal ethics is concerned with describing the dividing moral lines between the species and prescribing new ways of conceptualizing moral hierarchies (see, e.g., Fischer 2020), my interest lies in investigating the practitioners' experiences and ways of handling moral questions. Here, I turn to the anthropology of morality, which addresses people's moral striving in the context of reproduction, care, death, and dying (Gammeltoft 2014; Jackson 1998; Kaufman 2005; Lambek 2015; Mattingly 2014; Mol, Moser, and Pols 2010; Morgan 2009; Sharp 2019; Taylor 2017; Wahlberg 2018; Wool 2015). In particular, Cheryl Mattingly's work on moral laboratories (2014) and Lesley Sharp's study of the morality of human-animal encounters (2019) have been a crucial source of inspiration. Mattingly urges us to explore how people as experiencing subjects strive to live morally worthy lives (2014, 10) and how this striving is "marked with a radical uncertainty" (16). In this approach, studying morality is not so much about people's ideas of "the good." Rather, it focuses on how they face frailty, how they doubt, and how they strive to do good. Situated in animal laboratories, a field close to my own, Sharp's study unlocks the moral actions of professionals and suggests that we focus on the "wrestling associated with moral conundrums" (2019, 8) when care, suffering, and death of animals are inescapable. Following this approach, I wish to understand "morality-in-the-making" (Mesman 2008, 11) in "contexts marked by ambiguity, uncertainty, or incongruity" (Sharp 2019, 8). I examine how various professionals experience holding in trust the lives of animals and humans in their care and how they struggle to determine the worth of these beings. This may sometimes involve letting infants die, and in the Newborn Pig Facility it always involves putting down piglets, thus alerting us to the coexistence of care for both life and death in these settings.

My interest is not in morality per se, as is the case of most work within the anthropology of morality. Rather, I investigate how the moral experience shapes the way liminal lives are framed and constituted. I thus challenge the human-centeredness of the anthropology of morality and bring the moral dimension into conversation with multispecies ethnography. This conversation enables me to weave the complex attachments and detachments that make liminal lives gain or lose worth together with the moral quandaries of professional caregivers who try to find their way in the midst of unexpected circumstances. By investigating the role of moral experiences in constituting life, I engage the "uncanny interface" between multispecies ethnography focused on human-animal relations and the anthropology of morality interested in first-person human experiences.[13] As much as substitution is a result of distributed agency that unsettles boundaries, it also involves taking a moral stance; making judgments; and drawing boundaries among species, between life and death, and between belonging and not belonging in society.

BELONGING

The topic of belonging has been central to social scientists studying how reproductive technologies, policies, and practices involve the selection of lives (Gammeltoft 2014; Koch 2014; Morgan 2009; Murphy 2017; Rapp 1999; Roberts 2007; Scheper-Hughes 1992; Spalletta 2021; Stasch 2009; Wahlberg 2018). Likewise, scholarship on immigration has pointed to the ways in which immigration policies shape belonging by selecting among lives, among different forms of suffering, and between wanted and unwanted migrant subjects (Fassin 2018; de Leon 2015; Ticktin 2011). To my knowledge, no studies bring together the selection of human lives in the fields of reproduction and human migration, and not very many studies bring together the selection of human and animal lives in the same study.[14] This is what I do in this book. I argue that practices of substitution in the NICU, the animal facility, and immigration policies actualize the pivotal question of who and what belongs and involve letting particular kinds of lives into and out of society. By bringing these two fields together, I reveal connections between what appears at first sight to be the dissimilar life-and-death decisions in neonatology and practices of selection at Denmark's border policies.

Nira Yuval-Davis (2011) makes a distinction between belonging as an experience and belonging as a politics. In this book, I address only the latter meaning of belonging—that is, belonging as an exercise of power that delineates the boundaries of a collectivity and organizes who and what may or may not have membership. In the NICU, the clinicians used the term "attachment" (*tilknytning*) to describe the parents' bonding with their infant, and in that case, parents' attachment to their child often appeared as a moral imperative independent of the infant's chance of surviving (Navne, Svendsen, and Gammeltoft 2018). Moreover, as we saw in the case of Cheung's parents, parental attachment may also influence life-and-death decision making when an infant is on the verge of life. Where the "sixth IVF attempt" might move the child across the border of viability, parents who are hesitant about providing active treatment and forming an attachment to their child might move the child toward palliative care. In the discussion of Cheung's parents in the noon conference, their initial hesitant attachment led the clinicians to discuss the parents' national attachment to Denmark. The clinicians' concern about the survival of the individual child included a concern about the child's future life and attachment to his or her family and the welfare state. Here, national belonging became a question of whether the welfare state could expect to support a child.

In other cases I followed, decisions about whether and how to continue the various life-sustaining processes were intertwined with considerations about the state costs of supporting such a child through a lifetime and how a severely disabled child would be able to contribute to society. Practices of substituting for precarious infants actualized two border crossings—between life and death, and between belonging and not belonging in Denmark. In this book, I see the clinical orientation toward attachment to family and welfare state as a politics that shapes the inclusion and exclusion of particular precarious infants.

Substitution as a practice of societal inclusion and exclusion was also strongly present in the Newborn Pig Facility. When Marie and Thomas agree to end the life of piglet L, and when Peter and Anna try to figure out the situation of piglet R, their practices of substitution concern both the well-being of the individual piglets (Will it be possible to stabilize the animal and minimize its pain?) and the pigs' potential to improve nutrition for infants like Cheung (Will it be possible to turn the piglet into data that might contribute to good health for infants?). In these situations, substitution involves selecting which piglets are to enter, stay, or leave the experiment—selections that we may see as practices of making pigs join or leave a societal collectivity of pigs and people. In other words, for both humans and pigs, birth constitutes a passing into society, and for the professionals overseeing this passage, substituting for fragile bodies raises questions about who and what belong in society.

In Danish human immigration policies, the word "attachment" has come to play a crucial role. In 2000, the term "attachment requirement" (*tilknytningskrav*) was introduced in the Danish Aliens Act, forcing applicants to make themselves familiar with Danish history, language, and values. This represents an orientation toward the national community that may be conceptualized as an affective governmentality (Bissenbakker 2019, 181). At that time, Denmark was the first nation in Europe to use "national attachment" as a legal way to regulate family reunification. In contrast to the "discrete authority" of parental attachment in the NICU (Navne and Svendsen 2019), the "attachment requirement" in immigration law is publicly known and politicized. Despite these differences, in bringing together the two fields, I aim to understand the logics and ideas about familial and national belonging that regulate entry to society through birth and at geopolitical borders. At yet another border, pig's entry into Denmark at the geographical border between Denmark and Germany is also being regulated. In 2019, a wild boar fence was established at the Danish-German border to prevent wild boars in Germany from migrating into Denmark. As I show in chapter 4, bringing together measurements for regulating the entry of migrating humans and pigs alerts us to the intertwined processes of selection and care in practices of substitution.

In scrutinizing belonging as a politics that is about including and excluding not only different kinds of humans (infants and migrants) but also different kinds of pigs (wild boars and domestic pigs), I draw on Kregg Hetherington's concept of "agribiopolitics" (2020, 12) and Stefan Helmreich's concept of "symbiopolitics" (2009, 15).[15] Both concepts break with the humanist framework of Michel Foucault ([1976] 1990) by extending the "bio" in biopolitics to include relationships among humans, animals, microbes, and plants. While agribiopolitics refers to political techniques that make certain populations of humans thrive alongside populations of crops (Kregg Hetherington 2020, 13), symbiopolitics refers to governance practiced in semiotic and material entanglements between humans and nonhumans (Helmreich 2009, 15) beyond the agricultural field. Agribiopolitics guides my investigation of how human life and welfare in the Danish context are enabled by governing populations of pigs and crops. Symbiopolitics informs my attention to how the government of humans, animals, and crops that move into or out of Denmark enacts and shapes the welfare state collectivity. I use the term "welfare state collectivity" to designate an imagined collectivity of humans and nonhumans standing in a reciprocal relationship to the welfare state and seen as crucial to its preservation. This concept draws upon theories of imagined communities (see, e.g., Anderson 2006; Gullestad 2002; Schinkel 2017) and directs attention to how the governance of entangled beings enacts ideas about collectivity and what counts as belonging when it comes to humans, animals, and crops.

To understand the profundity of these questions in the Danish context, I next provide the historical background for understanding relationships among humans and pigs in this part of the world. I begin by scrutinizing the agribiopolitical relations, which made the human population thrive alongside pigs, and I then turn to the symbiopolitical relations at stake in the parallel management of pig and human procreation.

PIGS AND PEOPLE IN DENMARK

The Newborn Pig Facility is located on the campus of the Royal Veterinary and Agricultural University, which was founded in Copenhagen in 1856. At that time, the Danish population numbered two million people, 80 percent of whom lived in the countryside. The production of cereals for the British market made up a major source of income for the Danish nation. In the 1870s, as a response to declining cereal prices, many Danish farmers shifted to the production of animal products, a change that has been described as one of the greatest successes in the history of Danish business (Henriksen and Kærgård 2014; Kærgård 2017). In this new economy, the production of pork and butter increased significantly.[16] In the beginning of the twentieth century, Danish pork production was elevated to a national project, as a way to produce wealth for the nation and let the population thrive on the pig as a national economic resource.[17] The cooperative movement that emerged in Danish farming communities in the nineteenth century strongly shaped the Danish political system, and a strong alliance between the farming communities and the state was built, supported by all parties in the Danish Parliament. The Danish state came to play a significant role in facilitating the national coordination of pork production. In the first half of the twentieth century, the national economic importance of industrialized porcine life was indisputable, and Danish economic and foreign policy were sensitive to demands from the pork industry (Hansen 2002).

Breeding livestock is a way of intervening in the reproduction of a population to optimize economic profit. In the twentieth century, breeding programs resulted in the renowned Danish "bacon pig," which had a set of extra ribs, lean meat, and large litters and which constituted a steady source of income for Danish agriculture through the first half of the century. The Danish pig stock represented "breed wealth" (Franklin 2007, 107), a repository of genetic and reproductive capital on which the production depended.[18] Danish pig farming came to be organized in cooperatives united in what is now called the Danish Agriculture and Food Council, which is responsible for the national coordination of breeding, production, and export and has close connections to the political system.[19] Today, welfare for pigs in Danish barns is regulated by the state in alignment with European Union legislation and exercised in a way that combines care for animals and control of animals and farmers (Anneberg and Vaarst 2018, 99).[20] As the piglets from the refined Danish pig population enter the Newborn Pig Facility, selection of life is also inescapable in daily laboratory practices. Deciding on membership in the Danish pig resource at the farm and in the lab is an act of governing and constructing which pigs belong in Denmark.

During the more than 150 years that have passed since the opening of the Royal Veterinary and Agricultural University, the human population of Denmark has almost tripled, reaching 5.6 million, yet the share of humans living in rural areas has dropped from 80 percent in the middle of the nineteenth century to 3 percent at the beginning of the twenty-first century. In the same period, the annual number of pigs produced increased more than fifty times from half a million in the 1880s to twenty-six million in 2018. The increased productivity is due to mechanization and technical progress, in combination with structural changes that have led to fewer, larger, and more specialized farms (Pedersen, Schlægelberger, and Larsen 2018, 20–26). Despite the increase in animals, pig production today does not constitute the income to the country it used to. Where the agricultural sector contributed around 20 percent to the country's GDP in 1916, its contribution (of which pig production constitutes a large part) was around 2 percent in 2015 (Pedersen and Møllenberg 2016, 7) and the economic importance of pork continues to be a contested issue.

Today, 66 percent of Danish land is cultivated, which is among the world's most intense exploitation of the land in any country. On a sunny day from the window of an airplane going from one end of Denmark to the other—a flight of less than one hour—one will notice that almost all land is divided into fields of different colors, yet few people will recognize that fodder for pigs and other livestock is what is primarily grown on those fields.[21] The structure of this landscape is inextricably linked to the country's production of high-quality pork meat. Governing the pig population to generate wealth for humans is enabled by governing crops and their health. Despite their high number, the animals themselves are absent from view.[22] Driving through the countryside in Denmark, one rarely sees a single pig, and only insiders will recognize the presence of pigs when passing slurry tanks next to low-rise barns and fodder silos. The agribiopolitical relations shaping the Danish landscape and pig lives continue to raise public discussions of livestock's contribution to climate change and the pollution of Danish waters. During my years of research for this book, everyone I spoke to about Danish pork production acknowledged the key role it had played in the Danish economy in the nineteenth and twentieth centuries, and most people considered pork a basic food. Yet there was also embarrassment and concern about the pigs' environmental impact and their compromised welfare in barns.

Pride in national achievements related to Danish pig breeding, attention to the environment and animal welfare, and an ambition to create new career paths for pigs are all reflected in the history of the Royal Veterinary and Agricultural University. From the establishment of the university, applied biology has been key to educational and research activity there, and the university has had close relations with the meat producing industry. Yet through the twentieth century, new agendas for animal welfare, sustainable use of natural resources, and healthy agricultural products entered the national consciousness. By the end of the century, the institution engaged in research and provided education on all aspects of the production and consumption process from farm to gut, and it played a central role in the successes of Danish biotech companies and the country's pharmaceutical and food industries.[23] In 2005, the Royal Veterinary and Agricultural University became part of the Life Science Faculty at the University of Copenhagen, and in 2012, the majority of departments in this faculty were moved into the Faculty of Health Sciences. Later this faculty's veterinary departments constituted the School of Veterinary Medicine and Animal Science of which the Newborn Pig Facility is now part. These changes of names and organizational affiliations tell the story of a veterinary field that has moved closer to human bio-medicine by emphasizing commonalities between the shared biology of humans and animals and by participating in "One Health" initiatives.[24] Hence, the arrival of the unnamed piglets in the Newborn Pig Facility and Cheung in the human NICU are situated within a larger social arena of Danish agricultural develop-ments and advances in medical science and technology that have been brought together because of attention to a shared human-animal biology. In contrast to the United Kingdom and United States, there was never a strong antivivisection movement in Denmark. I see this absence as closely related to the growth of a national economy in which livestock became such an essential part of the human community's economic and national development.

The legislative and institutional framework of the lives of both pigs and people in Denmark is what in everyday language is called the welfare state (velfærdsstaten) or the welfare society (velfærdssamfundet). Like the state in the other Nordic countries, the Danish welfare state was established as part of the process of modernization. In the first half of the twentieth century, as a prag-matic response to the structural changes of industrialization and an increase in the supply of female labor, social reforms introduced first public health insur-ance, disability insurance, public nurseries, and care for the aged and later child support payment and old age pensions for all citizens (Christiansen and Petersen 2001). We might conceptualize this conglomerate of social reforms as an insti-tutionalization of substitution. For example, in 1949 the Danish Housewife Replacement Law introduced in-home care by state-employed caregivers, who stepped into the home and substituted for an absent or sick housewife. The name of the law suggested a kind of kinship, in which the state would replace some of its citizens. From the beginning, access to welfare benefits was based on citizenship and territorial belonging, and access to welfare benefits went hand in hand with a strong emphasis on financial independence, active participation in society, and individual self-determination. The welfare state was as much a moral project of making citizens enlightened (through providing education to every-one) and teaching them to act ethically (by paying taxes, respecting the laws, and taking responsibility for the community) as it was a bureaucratic one. Con-sequently, to most Danes, welfare does not refer to the possibility of living off government benefits through a lifetime. Rather, it involves active participation in society and connotes a mutual exchange between state and citizens. The indi-vidual has to strive for economic independence and pay taxes to the state, while the state has to redistribute goods. The individual has responsibilities, yet risk sharing is collectively distributed (O. Pedersen 2018, 69–73). This vision of the social contract between state and citizen includes the ideal that every citizen would contribute to realizing a collectivity in which every life was considered to be of equal worth and would put the community above the individual (O. Pedersen 2018, 59–65). Central principles were equality, solidarity, and universal access to welfare benefits (Merrild 2018). A caring and compassionate state based on principles of solidarity and the redistribution of tax revenue was to secure the social equality and individual autonomy of citizens within a reciprocally binding community (Bendixsen, Bringslid, and Vike 2018; Trägårdh 2010). Thus, what characterizes the Nordic countries is their equity-driven principle of universal benefits, according to which every resident (independent of their economic situation) is eligible for services. In this system of well-defined social rights, the state and nation appear as intrinsic to each other and in a close relationship to the people.[25]

In Denmark, the welfare state has largely positive connotations of a collectivity that residents are part of as both taxpayers and recipients of benefits. Compared to the situation in other countries, in Denmark differences between high and low incomes are relatively small, and the country's tax rate is one of the highest in the world (Danish Ministry of Taxation 2018). All residents have free access to health care throughout their lives, from prenatal care to care in the last stages of life. In addition to health care, the state subsidizes the cost of nurseries, schools, university education, and nursing homes and provides stipends for students and social benefits in case of unemployment, sickness, or retirement. Consequently, citizens live their lives in close association with state institutions, which most people see as trustworthy partners as well as self-evident platforms within which they are born, mature, acquire knowledge and skills, receive care, and eventually die.

Since the late 1980s, neoliberal incursions have dominated welfare state politics[26] and turned the prioritization of welfare state resources into one of the most central political battlefields in Danish politics (Magnussen, Vrangbæk, and Saltman 2009). This focus on prioritizations has been part of governmental reasoning that makes citizens' access to welfare state resources dependent on their moral behavior and alignment with the norms of the welfare state (Bengtsson, Frederiksen and Larsen 2015; Spalletta 2021). Moreover, the orientation toward prioritization has drawn into question the need to provide services to people in precarious positions, in particular individuals at the margins of or outside the labor market and newly arrived non-Western immigrants (J. Andersen 2019). For example, in the 2010s, Denmark's laws about immigration were tightened and benefits were cut for people arriving from countries outside the European Union, turning Denmark into an anti-immigration hardliner among European nations—a change also reflected in the use of the "attachment requirement" as a juridical tool to reduce immigration (Bissenbakker 2019, 188). Stricter immigration laws have challenged the idea of the welfare state collectivity as equivalent with the national territory, as cuts in benefits to asylum seekers in the country illustrate what Marry-Anne Karlsen refers to as "a growing willingness to distinguish between people based on hierarchies of worth" (2018, 239).

Welfare state regulations and institutions also shape which pigs and people are born. In chapter 1, I describe the Danish history of pig breeding, and in chapter 3, I provide a history of Danish human reproductive health policies, but here I briefly mention the case of assisted human reproduction and prenatal screening to illustrate how symbiopolitical relations among pigs and humans shape who and what come to belong in the welfare state collectivity. As part of extensive reproductive health care in Denmark, state-financed IVF is subsidized for all women regardless of marital status and sexual self-identification,[27] which constitutes one of the world's most liberal provisions of fertility treatment. In 2019, 9.2 percent of all births in Denmark resulted from fertility treatment (The Danish Health Data Authority 2021, 10). As the use of IVF creates a higher risk of preterm birth, the political support for IVF as a way of building families is, thus, closely related to the clinical work in the NICU, also reflected in Dr. Karen's attention to the procreative history of the Chinese couple. The liberal state-subsidized access to IVF in Denmark reflects the political view that the good citizen is a reproductive citizen (Mohr and Koch 2016) and that having children is a way of becoming a full person and gaining membership in a procreative welfare state collectivity (Tjørnhøj-Thomsen 2005). Despite the great differences between the regulation of pig breeding and human reproduction, both fields rely on assisted reproductive technologies. The shared ambition of procreative futures for both pigs and humans results in some of the world's largest litters among pigs and most liberal access to IFV among humans. Moreover, although the regulation of human reproduction differs greatly from the forced insemination of sows, selection is present in both fields. In pig breeding, selection is a means of genetically upgrading a herd and excluding less favored traits from it. In human prenatal diagnostics, selection takes place in webs of kinship and involves increased attention to chromosomal and genetic disorders. For example, in 2004 Denmark became the first country in the world to introduce state-financed screening for Down syndrome. Uptake was high (above 95 percent), which resulted in a marked drop in the number of infants born with the syndrome.[28] Consequently, the pronatalist commitment in pig and human reproductive politics coexists with governmental efforts to prevent particular individuals from being born. The Danish regulation of the reproduction of pigs and humans embodies what Ayo Wahlberg and Tine Gammeltoft refer to as a shift from assisted reproductive technologies "helping nature" to selective reproductive technologies "guiding nature" and preventing particular kinds of neonates from being born (2018, 4–5). In pig breeding, "guiding nature" has become thoroughly institutionalized. In human reproductive policies, "helping nature" is dominant in IVF treatments, whereas "guiding nature" has a presence in prenatal diagnostics. Moreover, as the case of Cheung shows, despite the pronatalist ambition of saving premature infants, selection is an inescapable question in life-and-death decision making. Viewed together, pig and human reproductive policies delineate who and what has membership in the welfare state collectivity.

The concepts of agribiopolitics and symbiopolitics invite us to explore complex intersections among entangled beings. In this book, I begin with intersections between pigs and people, yet I extend these relationships to crossings of humans, animals, and crops in and out of Denmark. In bringing together, on the one hand, life-and-death decision making in the Newborn Pig Facility and the human NICU and, on the other hand, crossings of agricultural products and animal and human immigrants, I explore how substitution practices involve selecting not only what people and things are allowed inside Denmark, but also which people are seen as appropriate for state support. My argument is that the selection of lives—be it in connection with birth or the geographical border—is directly linked to ideas about sustaining equal life opportunities and high levels of universal care for humans who have already been let into the welfare state. To phrase it differently, the exclusion of lives in agriculture, animal experiments, human medicine, and migration policies brings to the fore strong notions of equity. The widespread Danish norm of aiming for equal access to health care and high standards of living for everyone involves selecting who is to be included in the collectivity. While Denmark is often portrayed as a thoroughly equalitarian society, *Near Human* exposes the practices of differentiating between lives that are woven into the visions and practices of social equity in the Danish context. Differentiating is a powerful tool of forming borders. As Marianne Lien, Heather A. Swanson, and Gro B. Ween remind us, "marginality (like periphery) is constantly made, enacted by narratives as well as practices" (2018, 3). By focusing on how borders are produced in substituting for human and animal lives, I show that borders and border crossers are not marginal to the welfare state, but rather are at the center of defining which species and which forms of life belong in Denmark.

COLLABORATIVE RESEARCH

The research on which this book is based has been thoroughly collaborative and took place between 2009 and 2019. In 2009, when Lene Koch and I embarked on the Pig Project, a research project about the pig as a model of the human, I contacted the research director of the Newborn Pig Facility, Professor Per Torp Sangild (hereafter, "Professor Per"). He was excited by the fact that his pig facility—not only the human clinic—was worth the attention of a medical anthropologist. He saw me as a possible partner in his pioneering endeavor of making his pig studies of interest to human neonatologists. In introducing me and later Mie Seest Dam, one of my graduate students, to his collaborating partners, he often referred to us as "the social scientists who help us translate our pig studies

into the clinic." He thereby situated his research in the field of translational medicine, a field that has become increasingly important in biomedical research and
funding landscapes. In particular, comparisons between experimental animals
and human patients have been advocated anew as a critical component of taking
research from the bench to the bedside.

My initial fieldwork in the Newborn Pig Facility paved the way for my engagement in the research platform NEOMUNE (a combination of the words "neonate" and "immune") which ran between 2013 and 2019. NEOMUNE was funded
through a prestigious grant from Innovation Fund Denmark, a state-financed
agency, to establish a research platform in which studies in piglets and mice were
coupled with observational and clinical studies in NICUs in several countries.
Taking seriously the translational ambition, NEOMUNE research aimed at
developing new diet and microbiota treatments for normal and compromised
newborn infants and of establishing adequate and universally accepted clinical
care procedures for infants with limited access to mother's milk. In particular,
NEOMUNE sought to translate raw milk—that is, colostrum—from Danish
dairy cows into the guts of preterm infants in the NICU. To reach this objective,
NEOMUNE incorporated the whole process, from laboratory studies through
clinical studies to marketable nutrition products commercially sold to NICUs
or parents globally. A central aspect of realizing this translational ambition was
the enrollment of partners from universities, hospitals, and the dairy industry
along with a "spatialization of experiment" (Murphy 2017, 79), which involved
gaining access to infant populations and building infrastructures for collaboration and data generation by setting up clinical studies in Denmark and China.
NEOMUNE included a small social science work group, which focused specifically on translational processes between experimental and clinical research.
Heading this study, I (along with Mie) became part of the NEOMUNE team for
six years, collaborating with the researchers and clinicians involved in taking care
of piglets, data, and infants.

During my years of engagement with the Newborn Pig Facility, I followed the
transition of the research group, which began by running experiments in a win-
dowless basement with concrete floors and walls and homemade incubator
boxes and built a new and much larger facility with new equipment and technology on the ground floor of the same building. Concurrently, the studies
expanded from focusing on how specific forms of nutrition such as cow colostrum prevent necrotizing enterocolitis to increasingly approaching the body as a
whole (in contrast to separate organs within it) and studying the gut-brain connection. Reflecting the inrush of prestige and funding to the Newborn Pig Facility, this transition points to a political landscape for research that encourages
partnerships across public universities and private companies, across Asia and
Europe, across agriculture and biomedicine, and across animals and humans.
While the research I followed in Professor Per's group used pigs as models for

human infants, he always thought of translation as movements in both directions across life science, agriculture, and the clinic.

In 2013 I initiated a five-year social science project (called the LifeWorth project) on negotiations of life and its worth at the beginning and end of life, a project that was realized through funding from the Danish Council for Independent Research. LifeWorth and NEOMUNE made it possible for me to continue my collaboration with Lene and employ three graduate students—Mie, Laura Emdal Navne, and Iben Mundbjerg Gjødsbøl—who did extensive fieldwork in research, clinical, and care sites and with whom I have carried out interviews, shared fieldwork data, and worked closely in all respects. Between 2013 and 2018, these four people were my fieldwork companions, guides, and discussion partners. In the last year of the LifeWorth project I employed Anja Bornø Jensen, an associate professor who investigated the pigs' role in integrating the lab and the clinic in the field of organ transplantation and introduced me to important new sites for the use of pigs in translational medicine. Most of the thoughts in this book are a testimony to the shared reflections of the LifeWorth group and our practice of moving between different sites of care for life at the edge.[29]

In the Newborn Pig Facility and the human NICU, my most important source of insight comes from episodic fieldwork conducted between 2009 and 2014. During fieldwork I followed researchers and clinicians as they performed their daily tasks, conducted formal interviews with the various professional groups in both settings, and engaged in many informal conversations, as well as participating in seminars and workshops related to translating animal-based knowledge into clinical practice. In addition, between 2013 and 2019, I attended eight large NEOMUNE symposia (in Denmark and abroad), went on a short trip with NEOMUNE researchers to China to engage with collaborating NICU partners, and visited the Danish company that produced cow colostrum and dairy farmers who had contracts with it. I also visited a conventional Danish pig farm. Concurrently, Lene and I researched the use of nonhuman primates in Danish laboratories, a study I return to in chapter 2 as a case I juxtapose to the use of pigs. In this book, my own fieldwork experiences are complemented by Mie's ethnography from the Newborn Pig Facility in 2013 and Laura's ethnography from the human NICU in 2014, both of which I draw on.[30] My empirical material also includes a wide range of policy documents and newspaper articles in relation to pork production, animal-based human medicine, preterm infants, and migration into Denmark.

Although I apply the term "multispecies" to my work, humans remain squarely in the foreground. While I am sensitive to the world of pigs, I do not attempt to understand what it is to be pig or to write about the world from a perspective that gives equal space to humans and animals. In entering livestock farms or observing, feeding, and attending to piglets in experimental science, I have mainly followed my human (speaking) informants in their engagements with animals rather than practiced etho-ethnography.[31] In the human NICU, I encountered and talked with the parents but did not explicitly explore the parental experience, and I did not pursue an interest in infant personhood. My primary concerns were to attend to the daily routines of neonatal care and to observe the formal and informal discussions regarding treatment strategies in relation to infants at the margins of life.

While this book grows out of my collaboration with members of the Life-Worth team, multidisciplinarity is an equally fundamental condition for my research. Without the collaboration of biomedical researchers and clinicians and their openness to perspectives beyond those of natural science, this book would not exist. Professor Per generously welcomed anyone into his group who took an interest in its work. He was exemplary in the way he connected a variety of actors to the pig studies, stayed curious about other people's perspectives, respected their experiences and views, and always demonstrated an admirable enthusiasm for collaboration and facilitating a strong spirit of teamwork. The head of the NICU, Dr. Mads, showed the same kind of interest in social science perspectives and invited me in, without putting restrictions on the activities I could follow. I benefited tremendously from this openness to the world. Nevertheless, our collaboration has not been without tensions. Professor Per's statement about the social scientists helping the natural scientists in translating pig studies into better health for infants is a statement that identifies my cultural expertise as a kind of derivative, which comes after the fact. From this perspective, science is purified from culture but meets culture when scientific facts are to be translated into society—a translation that requires cultural competences from the anthropologist. Scholarship in anthropology and science and technology studies over the past thirty years contests this perspective on the relationship between science and society (Franklin 2007; Haraway 1997; Keller 1992; Latour and Woolgar 1979; Mol 2002) and argues that what social scientists need to explore is how the laboratory is conditioned by society and how the laboratory conditions society. During the years of my collaboration with people at the Newborn Pig Facility and the human NICU, Professor Per's straightforward statement about social scientists assisting natural scientists has been accompanied by discussions between us about how laboratory life may be studied by social scientists and how to collaborate.

In inhabiting these collaborative relations across epistemological differences, the concept of "critically engaged research" (Svendsen 2009, 38) has helped me address the double roles my biomedical colleagues and I had to navigate. As an anthropologist, I was inclined to critically address the dominant assumptions of the field of translational medicine and refuse "to accept immediate, common-sense understanding, while at the same time having the most profound respect for and curiosity about commonsense understandings" (Frank 2010, 73). But as a colleague of my biomedical researchers—sharing NEOMUNE funding with them—I wished to engage the challenges and concerns they faced. This engagement was grounded in direct interactions and solidary relationships with my colleagues in the biomedical fields.

In entering peer-like relationships with the researchers and clinicians, I shared my findings with them, always inviting them to read and comment on my papers before publication. This exchange of papers and the discussions that followed spelled out to me not only the epistemological differences between us, but also the fact that we wanted to know different things that were not always experienced as compatible. My collaborative experiences in translational medicine illuminate that moving between the bench and the bedside is not only a question of ferrying knowledge from one species (pigs) to another species (humans) and vice versa. Rather, translation involves discussions about what counts as knowledge and thus implies translation between disciplinary "species."

Critically engaged scholarship is rarely a smooth experience. It can be unsettling for the biomedical researcher to be an object of the gaze of the anthropologist, and it can be an unsettling experience for the anthropologist to conduct critical research while entering joint relationships with one's colleagues and hosts in the biomedical field. More than anything, I acquired a sensitivity to and alertness about the boundary practices at stake in the open-door politics of the animal facility. What was legitimate knowledge in the space of the laboratory (articulations of pigs as almost patients or kin) may appear not only misplaced, but also threatening in public spaces such as conferences and scientific articles. The spatial politics of knowledge has been masterfully researched in anthropology (see, for example, Geissler 2013; Jain 2010). Less thematized are the ways in which solutions to the ethical challenges of that spatial politics are worked out in multidisciplinary research collaborations. In teaching qualitative methodology and research ethics to public health students concurrently with conducting fieldwork and writing papers, I have come across very little work that addresses the ethics of writing. In contrast, ethical guidelines focusing on access to the field and interaction with informants are abundant. In my close collaboration with highly esteemed professionals in the biomedical field, ethical questions about what can go into the analysis have been my steady companions. Self-censorship has always been lying in wait, ready to sneak up on me and challenge me to find a way of writing that could be critical and engaged at the same time and not cause trouble in collaborative relations.

Most likely, I was not the only one who found that collaborative relationships in NEOMUNE questioned the common sense of the production of knowledge. As basic science and clinical researchers from diverse environments and different parts of the world interfaced and collaborated, all of us were—more or less—on foreign territory and had to find our footing and navigate our way. More than once, some of the researchers in the Newborn Pig Facility teasingly asked Mie and me, "Okay, so we are your piglets?" In jokingly describing themselves as our pigs (belonging to another—disciplinary—species), they hinted at the ways in which they were both our colleagues (of equal standing) and our empirical resources (of unequal standing) in the multispecies collaboration in which we all participated. Afterwards, Mie and I would joke that if they were our pigs, they were certainly free-range. Our joking not only expressed the readiness to cross from the human to the pig and the unattractive position of the pig, which is pulled and pushed by forces that are more powerful than it is, but it also illustrated that both sides experienced a loss of control (by being a resource of another knowledge practice or by being unable to tame free-range animals). Nevertheless, a mutual willingness to collaborate and engage with each other's perspectives has survived and strengthened our collaborations. It has also resulted in a few coauthorships (Dam et al. 2017; Dam, Sangild, and Svendsen 2018; Dam, Sangild, and Svendsen 2020), which represent an action of translation and a striving for socially robust scholarship readable by and of interest to both natural scientists and social scientists.

In this book I propose that in multispecies collaboratives, the value of social science lies in empirically exploring the contamination between humans and animals along with the boundary work that continuously divides and connects the spaces, temporalities, and relations in which piglets and humans are allowed to act. In literally moving between the domains of humans and those of pigs, my ethnography is grounded in the daily interactions of people who think, feel, act, doubt, and negotiate at the same time as it seeks to explore these worlds by examining the logics that not only belong to them but encompass many of us. From this puzzled position we may begin to understand how human and animal lives create the conditions of possibility for one another.

THE ORGANIZATION OF THE BOOK

Near Human is organized around three border zones. Chapter 1 focuses on the borders between species. Chapters 2 and 3 focus on the borders between life and death. Chapter 4 focuses on the border between belonging and not belonging in the welfare state. In the ethnography of each chapter, I bring in social and historical context, thus adding layers of social context as the book progresses.

Chapter 1 explores the practices of feeding and follows cow colostrum from the farm to the Newborn Pig Facility and ultimately the human NICU. Theoretically, the chapter engages enactments of species boundaries and interspecies kinship in substitution practices. First, I trace the connections between experiments in the Newborn Pig Facility and Denmark's heritage of pig breeding and pork production, focusing on the development of cow colostrum as a feeding solution to prevent high mortality among newborn piglets. Second, I follow this feeding solution into the NICU via studies on piglets in the Newborn Pig Facility.

Here, treating the piglet as substitute for the infant shows the interspecies kinship between human and animal neonates through life-giving substances. Stepping closer to these kinship processes, I show that an anxiety about species belonging comes to the fore among researchers in the Newborn Pig Facility and parents in the human NICU. For both parties, invisiblizing interspecies kinship becomes an effective way of recognizing the human and situating it in intraspecies kinship.

Chapter 2 ethnographically enters the sacrificial exchange in ordinary laboratory routines and unfolds how piglets come into this world as substitutes for humans, at the same time as the piglets are themselves in need of substitution. Here, I bring multispecies ethnography and laboratory studies into a conversation with the anthropology of morality, thus highlighting how moral experience shapes the lives and deaths of piglets. I show that killing does not interrupt interspecies kinship but constitutes it. I end the chapter by situating the use of pigs in science in the history of the use of other research animals, particularly nonhuman primates. While these primates were used extensively in biomedical research throughout the twentieth century, by the end of that century in Europe it had become increasingly morally unpleasant to use them in research. I argue that the default identity of the pig as a killable animal provides the pig with flexibility. It can be turned into intimate kin in experimental practices and expendable animal on the day of dissection. Thus, upholding firm species boundaries between the original human and the pig substitute paves the way for the pig substitute to move across species boundaries in experimental practices.

Chapter 3 steps into the NICU and investigates life-and-death decision making. In following the cases in which clinicians express doubts about continued treatment, the chapter illuminates how substitution practices unsettle the border between life and death and involve decisions on who enters the welfare state. I discuss the social, temporal, and spatial imaginaries that come to the fore in substituting for infants and making decisions about continuing or withdrawing treatment. Drawing upon examples from the Newborn Pig Facility in chapters 1 and 2, I show that for both piglets and infants, relationships with the Danish welfare state are crucial in life-and-death decision making. While a meaningful life for the research piglet is defined as providing good data for the welfare state in the far future, in the NICU, happy family lives and reciprocal relationships to the welfare state in the near future are key markers for professionals who navigate these decision-making spaces. I ask why a readiness to discontinue treatment exists in a country in which every citizen is entitled to universal health services and social support. I answer this question by unraveling reproductive politics from the 1930s to the present, demonstrating that the exclusion of certain unborn lives has been part and parcel of welfare state politics focusing on inclusion and equality for nearly a century.

Chapter 4 takes researchers' ambition to transport pig-based knowledge and cow colostrum to NICUs in China as the empirical starting point for investigating how substitution practices unsettle geographical borders. First, I discuss the open gates that allow animal products, such as cow colostrum, to leave for China as part of sustaining a renowned Danish agricultural production. Second, I discuss Denmark's closed gates for wild boars and human migrants. Whereas the risk of wild boars infecting Danish pigs with African swine fever makes wild boars highly unwanted, the risk of migrants not contributing to society and becoming too costly for the state increasingly positions them as a threat to Denmark—thus demonstrating how the ecologically and demographically undesirable come together. By focusing on policies that determine who and what may cross Danish national borders, I show how Denmark is imagined as a metabolic organism that can take in only what is valuable and must keep out what is considered contaminating. Practices of substitution play a critical role in this metabolic thinking by identifying who can stand in for original Danes and who cannot. Substitution practices expose the coexistence of entanglements and border work and suspend a clear distinction between instrumental and intrinsic worth. Shifting the analytical attention from "what it means" to "what it takes" reveals how human and society come into being at the edges of life.

1 · FEEDING

Cows, Pigs, and Humans in Interspecies Kinship

Multiple births were inescapable when sows underwent cesarean sections in the Newborn Pig Facility. Usually, between eighteen and twenty-five piglets were transferred from the uterus of a sow to the incubator room. Here, individual incubator-like boxes—each containing a piglet—stood next to each other. On a shelf above, each incubator had a small machine that contained the liquid food and dispensed it by pushing it through a tube and into the catheter of the piglet. Despite the fact that the piglets came from the same litter, their common origin and siblingship were rarely expressed. In contrast, the connection between piglet and researcher was articulated to a much greater extent, often in lighthearted kinship terms.

One day in 2009, when I entered the Newborn Pig Facility to take part in feeding the piglets delivered by cesarean section a few days earlier, Rikke, the animal technician on duty, commented with a smile, "you are almost a part of the family now." This wording jokingly articulated a kin relationship between team members that included the anthropologist. On another day in the facility in 2013, Mie Seest Dam, one of my graduate students, drew gently heated milk into a plastic syringe and was about to feed the piglets when Thomas entered. "So you are the *madmor* today," he noted with a smile.[1] In Danish, *madmor* literally means "food mother." The concept originated in preindustrial rural Denmark, when the wife of the owner of a large traditional farm cooked for the servants living at the farm. When Thomas referred to Mie as *madmor*, he was referring to the piglets not so much as resources to be consumed (as pork or research data), but as members of the household (the farm) to be taken care of, as part of their belonging to and active participation in the research production.

The spatial dimensions of the experimental practices underpinned this notion of a shared household. The same building housed the Newborn Pig Facility on the first floor and the researchers' offices on the second floor. The researchers on duty "downstairs with the pigs" (meaning in the incubator room) would walk between the two floors many times a day, attending to the piglets and feeding them downstairs, running upstairs for a cup of coffee in the kitchen or to deal with email in the office, and then going downstairs again. By being installed in their incubators, the piglets were moved into the family of the researchers. In this sense the very setup of the experiment involved a "domesticatory practice" (N. Russell 2007, 40) in which the piglets could jokingly be treated, in line with the servants at the traditional farm, as an indispensable part of the family,[2] as we also saw in Thomas's humorous comment about the piglets as the team's "children."

In the Newborn Pig Facility, researchers based their experiments on the notion that premature pigs are biologically similar to premature human infants, and research protocols modeled care practices in the neonatal intensive care unit (NICU). Thus, most experiments called for the delivery of piglets 10–12 days before the sow was due (at 90 percent gestation). The researchers estimated that the physiology of these premature piglets is comparable to that of premature infants born in week twenty-seven (70–75 percent gestation), a delivery time that increases the risk of developing the inflammatory bowel disease necrotizing enterocolitis (NEC). The researchers' estimates are based on a long tradition of using pigs as models,[3] which has resulted in a huge literature documenting the anatomical and physiological similarities between human and pig (Bendixen et al. 2010; Bollen, Hansen, and Alstrup 2010; Dalgaard 2014; Gutierrez et al. 2015; Kuzmuk and Schook 2011; Miller and Ullrey 1987; Swindle et al. 2012; Sullivan et al. 2001; Sangild et al. 2014). In the 2000s, the mapping of the swine genome—an endeavor initiated by a collaboration between Danish and Chinese researchers—pointed out the great similarity between human and pig at the cellular level and proclaimed the "potential of the pig as a biomedical model" (Groenen et al. 2012, 393). In the Newborn Pig Facility, this biological proximity between human and pig made the pig an ideal animal in which to study the pathogenesis of gastrointestinal diseases in the perinatal period. By modeling the development of NEC in piglets, the researchers aimed to study the possible preventive effects of different forms of nutrition. The overall aim of the studies was to understand maturation of the gut and develop better nutrition for pre-term infants deprived of their mother's milk.

For the research team, the many similarities between human and pig documented in the scientific literature became a platform for treating the research piglets as the same "kind" as human infants born in the third trimester of pregnancy. The piglets replaced infants as research subjects and became "generic proxies" (Sharp 2014, 46). In being "generic," each piglet represented a nonspecific common biology and stood in for every other piglet in the experiment. In being "proxy," the pig replaced the human due to their biological relatedness. This notion of the same kind was emphasized in the research protocol, which used "neonate" or "mammalian fetus," terms that were not specific to either species and emphasized their similar biology.

In 2013, Professor Per established the NEOMUNE research platform. In line with his previous studies, the NEOMUNE studies treated piglet and infant as being of the same kind and ordered relations between them in terms of age. The studies investigated how cow colostrum affected gut maturation, growth, and neurodevelopment and prevented against NEC. Colostrum, the first milk produced after birth, is a rich source of proteins. In stimulating the immune system, colostrum facilitates the neonatal transition from the sterile fetal environment to the microbe-rich environment outside the uterus, which all mammals have to adapt to at birth. Colostrum is known for its protective qualities and life-giving nourishment and is referred to as "precious drops" or "liquid gold."[4] When infants are born prematurely, they are often deprived of a full diet of mother's milk (including colostrum), as premature birth makes it difficult to stimulate milk production. Professor Per believed that experiments documenting the positive outcome of using cow colostrum in piglets might predict positive effects of using cow colostrum in human infants.

This way of thinking suggested that maturity and life stage, rather than species, could be the relevant way to compare piglets and infants, as well as cow milk and human milk. It seemed possible that if colostrum produced by a cow could be fed with good results to premature pigs, it would be not only safe for premature infants (because other premature beings thrive on it), but also more suitable for a premature infant than mature human donor milk. In Denmark, as in a number of other countries, when mothers of preterm infants are unable to start breast-feeding or provide a full diet for their children, infants born before thirty-four weeks of gestation are fed human donor milk. This milk is produced by women who have been breast-feeding for at least a month. What Professor Per hypothesized was that cow colostrum—rather than human donor milk—would be the optimal diet for premature infants who did not have access to mother's milk during their first days of life. Infants deprived of "precious drops" from their own mother could instead be fed by the equivalent from a cow.

The colostrum studies set up a three-species relationship among cows producing colostrum on dairy farms, pigs standing in for infants in the experimental practices, and infants being fed cow colostrum tested on premature piglets. In this setup, cow colostrum became a less alien form of nutrition than human donor milk, and a cow that had newly given birth became closer kin to the infant than unfamiliar human mothers who had given birth several weeks earlier. The results of the pig studies showed that cow colostrum was as effective as human donor milk in protecting against NEC and was superior to both human donor milk and infant formula in stimulating growth, gut immunity, and digestive functions in premature piglets (M. Jensen et al. 2013; Støy et al. 2014; Rasmussen et al. 2016).

Based on these promising results, NEOMUNE initiated a randomized controlled pilot study that, for the first time in history, introduced cow colostrum to NICU infants born in gestational weeks 27–32. The study included premature infants from NICUs in both Denmark and China, who were fed spray-dried, reconstituted colostrum from Danish cows as a supplement to standard feeding.[5]

In the pilot study, the Newborn Pig Facility became a site of substitution and translation. As experimental subjects, piglets became substitutes for extremely premature infants at risk for developing NEC, and colostrum from dairy cows substituted for human milk if mothers had difficulty starting breast-feeding. By letting the piglets absorb cow colostrum and subsequently killing the piglets to study the colostrum's effects on their bodies, the researchers translated cow colostrum from the farm to the NICU. Translation means "carrying across" and refers to the linguistic process of transferring the meaning of a text from one language to another, a process that always involves a transformation of the original meaning. In this case, the first milk from the dairy cow was to be turned into small, handy ten-gram packages of spray-dried colostrum to be dissolved in cooled boiled water and fed through a tube to a premature infant. One such infant was Amanda. Her mother, Sofie, was in her thirtieth week of pregnancy when her water broke. Amanda was born nine weeks preterm and weighed 1575 grams. During Sofie's hospitalization, before she gave birth to Amanda, she and her husband were presented with the opportunity to participate in the NEOMUNE randomized controlled pilot study, which meant feeding Amanda cow colostrum as a supplement for the first two weeks of her life. The parents were a little nervous because it was the first time that cow colostrum would be used in a human infant trial, but in a conversation a few months after the birth, they emphasized their conclusion that cow colostrum is the closest you can come to a mother's own first milk. Sofie said: "I thought it was a good alternative. It was a bit strange, though, and we called her 'our little calf,' but there wasn't more in it than that. I think it [cow colostrum] is natural."[6]

Kin and kind often mutate in the context of reproductive technologies, as Donna Haraway notes (2008, 150). Sofie's joking embracement of a kinship connection to the cow and Thomas's amusing comments about the piglets being part of the family illuminate how different kinds become kin via cow colostrum's substituting for mother's milk and piglets' substituting for preterm infants. How is kinship part of translating cow colostrum from the farm to the NICU? In the process, what boundaries are crossed, erased, or created? What assumptions about humanity, animality, and use come to the fore in the technical and instrumental arrangement of replacing one species and substance for another?

In answering these questions, I follow cow colostrum at the farm, in the Newborn Pig Facility, and in the NICU and uncover how practices of substitution facilitate translation by emphasizing or de-emphasizing interspecies kinship. I argue that acts of disposal play a central role in materializing substitution and making cows, pigs, and humans eat from the same source and become kin. Yet concurrently, invisibilizing this interspecies kinship and upholding differences between kinds is essential to realizing bench-to-bedside translation. Consequently, as much as the erasure of species boundaries is part of what it takes to become a viable biographical life in the NICU setting, so too is the erection of species boundaries.

INTERSPECIES KINSHIP

In my conversations with researchers in the Newborn Pig Facility, the evolutionary connectedness between humans and pigs was spelled out to me again and again. In particular, the similarities between the gut of the pig and the gut of the human were central to the researchers' experiments, and thus biological kinship between pig and human—also central to the notion of the pig as a generic proxy—informed their vision of carrying cow colostrum from the farm through the lab to the clinic. Researchers outside the Newborn Pig Facility also emphasized the biological continuities between human and pig. In the field of organ transplantation, a research coordinator in charge of experimental studies with pigs told Anja Bornø Jensen and me: "The pig's similarity to the human is incredible. If you have a heart from a human and a heart from a pig in your hands, you cannot tell the difference." When I talked to senior scientists working with pig models, I noticed that treating the pig as biological kin was also part of their professional upbringing. They were part of a genealogy of scientists working with pigs and were now in the midst of training a new generation of researchers to use pigs as research animals (A. Jensen and Svendsen 2020).

Professor Per mentioned to me that he found the pig an attractive biomedical model for the human because in infancy the two species were similar not only in biology but also in terms of their color, size, and behavior. In his experience, piglets prompted and responded to care in the same way that human infants did. Moreover, I noticed that every researcher, regardless of academic age or background, would mention a kind of relatedness that transcended the biological: namely, the historical, national, and economic relations between pigs and humans—what Charis Thompson refers to as "animal use positions" (2013, 210). Thomas said, "when you have grown up eating meat and drinking milk and eating eggs, then it is just part of your culture." Here, the "it" that is "part of your culture" refers to the use of pigs (and other animals) as resources for humans, and the word also hints at an intimate knowledge of farm animals and farm products. As Sara Ahmed reminds us in her exploration of the meanings of use, use "gives us a sense of things: how they are; what they are like" (2019, 21). Among the researchers, using pigs produced feelings of familiarity and nearness.

Many of the researchers in the Newborn Pig Facility were veterinarians, and to many of them, the close connection between farming and research was part of their personal biography. Professor Per, for instance, was brought up on a pig farm, and this was also the case with a number of other researchers in the Newborn Pig Facility, including Thomas. In addition, several researchers who had not been brought up on a farm had spent their childhood years in rural parts of Denmark and had grandparents and other family members who were farmers. The theme of "going home to Jutland" (where the majority of Danish farming is located) for a weekend visit or the Christmas holidays was part of interactions in the laboratory. Thomas's amusing comment about Mie being *madmor* illustrates how the researchers continually went beyond the confines of the laboratory, bringing in the agricultural context, linking present lab practices to a history of farming, and jokingly treating the piglets as kin with whom they shared not only biology but also intimate living.

My conversations with the researchers about the background of and rationales for using pigs as models for humans suggest a relatedness between human and pig in terms of evolutionary connectedness, as well as the researchers' life-long familiarity with pigs as farm animals and hands-on experience with handling and caring for pigs in a laboratory context. The concept of relatedness is central to kinship studies in anthropology. Introduced by Janet Carsten and taken up by numerous anthropologists in the context of the new reproductive and genetic technologies, the concept of relatedness paves the way for thinking about kinship as "indigenous ways of acting out and conceptualizing relations between people" (Carsten 1995, 224).[7] In this light, kinship is a social practice that produces and marks exclusions and inclusions (Hird 2004, 219). Accordingly, anthropological kinship studies do not privilege biological ties and procreation. Ethnography from around the world has illuminated the great variation in how kin relationships are conceptualized and practiced. From this perspective, Western ways of thinking of kinship as rooted in biology are not universal, but a specific cultural logic.[8] In line with Carsten, Marshall Sahlins suggests that we take kinship and relatedness to refer to "'a mutuality of being': people who are intrinsic to one another's existence" (2011, 2). In her rich study of human-animal interactions in the Himalayas, Radhika Govindrajan argues that "relatedness always already exceeds the human" (2018, 6). The comment about Mie being a *madmor* and caring for an multispecies household and Sofie's humorous remark about her daughter as "our little calf" hint at how a mutuality of being gains presence while differences between human and animal remain.

In the following, I do not limit myself to "relations between *people*" or to how "*people* . . . are intrinsic to one another's existence" (my emphasis). Guided by the researchers' narratives about evolutionary connectedness (procreation through time) and filiation (in spaces of the farm and the lab) and parents' ambiguous comments about the child becoming a calf, I unravel the forms of interspecies and intraspecies kinship at stake in translating substances and bodies of one kind of value into another. Substitution creates interspecies kinship, which in turn facilitates translation. Yet in the end, upholding boundaries between human and animal is essential to carrying cow colostrum from the farm to the clinic.

DANISH PIG BREEDING AND PORK PRODUCTION

The cow colostrum fed to piglets in the experiments I followed in the Newborn Pig Facility was produced by the small Danish nutrition company Biofiber-Damino (hereafter, "Biofiber"), directed by Gunner Jacobsen.[9] For thirty years, Biofiber has specialized in producing nonmedicated feed supplements for use in intensive livestock production, and more recently it has expanded its range of expertise to include dietary supplements for humans. All its products are produced at a plant in western Denmark. Here, the company has established its own dairy factory for the collection and processing of cow colostrum. By far the majority of the colostrum processed is sold to pig farmers, who use it to increase the number of animals who survive the first few critical days of life. It is a refined version of this product that the piglet studies in Copenhagen aim to move into the guts of NICU infants.

"You know," Gunner says, "colostrum is a waste product at the dairy farms. We have a person who drives around to all the farms and picks it up. It is a full-time job just collecting the colostrum." On this beautiful spring day in 2014, he and I are talking on the veranda of a seaside hotel outside Copenhagen, during a two-day meeting for all the partners in the newly initiated NEOMUNE research platform. The meeting, which we are participating in, has brought together a group of 60–70 people: scientists running the pig studies, clinicians from the NICU, and representatives from the Danish nutrition and formula industries. The day has been packed with presentations on the relationship between gut microbiota and brain development within the overall framework of translating studies on piglets and clinical studies on infants into marketable colostrum and microbiota products for infants worldwide. With Gunner's comment about colostrum as a waste product, the field of agriculture is brought into our conversation about cutting-edge life science. On the veranda, I am reminded of the close relation between Professor Per's vision of "fewer infections, good digestion, better cognition for infants" in his introductory speech at the meeting and the widespread use of cow colostrum in livestock as a solution to perinatal death. In Danish piggeries, perinatal death is closely connected to producing sows that give birth to large litters. Breeding efforts involve choices about different potential animals (Sandøe and Christiansen 2008, 149). Selecting some traits in animals implies the rejection of other traits. Throughout the twentieth century, Danish pig breeding was concerned with growth and body composition, resulting in pigs with leaner meat, extra ribs, and fifteen centimeters added to their length. In pork production, assisted reproductive technology is not an offer for the childless but part of industrialized and institutionalized breeding. In the latter half of the twentieth century, farmers moved away from natural reproduction to injecting refined semen directly into the sow. Artificial insemination was increasingly favored as a way to reach breeding goals that made pigs cope better with production systems. In the early 1990s, selection for reproductive output—litter size and maternity care—was introduced as an additional trait, resulting in litter sizes that are the highest in Europe.[10] While sows have only fourteen teats, they would give birth to 20–25 piglets.

In 2010, however, the pigs' way of responding to this form of domestication hit the news. A national newspaper announced that "Oversized Litters Cause Millions of Deaths in Piglets"[11] and revealed that 24.2 percent of all live piglets born in Danish farrowing pens died within the first days of life—totaling more than 20,000 piglets every day (L. Pedersen et al. 2010; Danish Ministry of Food, Agriculture and Fisheries 2012; Rutherford et al. 2011, 21). This high mortality rate was directly connected to the nation's highly systematic national pig breeding programs.[12] Since the 1990s, the large litters of the Danish sows had caused low birth weight, increased teat competition due to the sow's not having enough teats to accommodate the entire litter, and increased piglet mortality. In addition, the piglets were born less mature, a circumstance that may also be related to the lean tissue growth and the large litter size (Sangild et al. 2014). The litter hierarchy, which is established within the first day after birth, leaves the weaker piglets either without access to colostrum or with access to only the low-quality colostrum of the rear teats (Bollen, Hansen and Alstrup 2010, 9). In short, breeding efforts aimed at an efficient conversion of Danish pigs to human wealth have shaped reproduction in such a way that a significant number of pig bodies could not access and process sufficient food and thus were expelled from the production process.[13]

In the public debate that followed, the lives and deaths of piglets were seen not only as a concern for the individual farmer or farming organizations, but also as raising ethical issues for the welfare state. This way of locating the responsibility for animal welfare in the state apparatus reflects a Danish history of close connections between the agricultural field and the state. These connections are also evident in the fact that animal welfare, including the welfare of production animals, is the legal and political responsibility of the Ministry of Food and Agriculture.[14] For more than a century, state institutions have had a central role in shaping the flesh, genetic makeup, and lives of pigs (Anneberg and Bubandt 2016; Anneberg and Vaast 2018). The central role of politicians—some of them farmers themselves[15]—in the debate about piglet mortality underpinned the position that although death in the farrowing pens was not illegal, the dead piglets there were individuals that had not received sufficient protection from the welfare state. According to a spokesperson from the Conservative People's Party, "the government needs to interfere if the farmers don't do it themselves."[16] The many voices in the debate did not base their outrage on the biological relatedness between human and pig emphasized by the scientists in the Newborn Pig Facility in talking about the pig as a valuable model organism. Rather, the social and political commitments to fragile piglets were based on the notion of a welfare state in which everyone, pigs as well as humans, contributes to the collectivity and in turn is provided with various forms of protection.

Although the discussion unambiguously concerned production pigs in the agricultural sector, not pets in people's homes, the public debate was silent about the routine annual killing of twenty-six million pigs in Denmark, which has a human population of fewer than six million. The minister of justice found the "increase in deaths" in the pig production process "concerning."[17] Although one could argue that overall deaths in production have increased throughout the twentieth and twenty-first centuries due to the increased number of pigs produced in the country, this argument was absent from public discussion. The public debate implicitly relied on a distinction between uncontrolled death in the first days after birth and controlled and legitimate slaughter after six months, which was considered part of acceptable use relations that turned pigs into value for farmers and the welfare state. As Ahmed writes, "use keeps something . . . alive, such that not to use something is to lose something" (2019, 4). In pointing to death in the farrowing pen as ethically unacceptable, the spokesperson from the Conservative People's Party treated use as a societal duty and made an association between using pigs and keeping them alive. In one short article in the national newspaper *Politiken*, the introductory lines read, "a calculation reveals that every fifth piglet dies before the age of one year."[18] The "one year" is obviously a mistake, as all suckling pigs in the industry are slaughtered at six months, yet this slip of the pen—together with repeated statements about the unethical death rates— underlines how the debate ignored pigs' predictable and scheduled death. Consequently, the piglets appeared not so much as production animals to be killed at six months, but as lives (maybe even coresidents or kin) with more open futures. Death itself was framed as a welfare problem in need of political action.

In 1890, a Danish manual about pig production referred to the pig as a very "flexible animal."[19] More than a century after this observation, the pig's flexibility was proved not only in terms of biology, but also in terms of its attachments to political and social commitments—what David Schneider has called "codes for conduct" in the context of kinship (1980, 51). The controversy reveals how the particular use relations embedded in industrial pork production raised moral concerns in the case of newborn piglets dying in the farrowing pens and silenced the twenty-six million Danish pigs annually that survive the first days of life in industrial barns before they are killed at the slaughterhouse at the age of six months.

Long before the controversy about death in the farrowing pens hit the national news, high piglet mortality in industrialized farming sparked Biofiber's development of its most sold product: cow colostrum as a feed supplement to make fragile newborn piglets thrive in the absence of sufficient teats and heat in production systems. Later, Professor Per found that the immature piglets from pork production farms—a result of breeding efforts aimed at large litters, lean meat, and extra ribs via artificial insemination—were excellent models for weak infants at risk of NEC. A sow from the Danish pork production process was transferred from a farm outside Copenhagen to the university stables a few days before having a cesarean section, which began the experiments in the Newborn Pig Facility. Thus, experimentation and substitution in the Newborn Pig Facility stand on an agricultural lineage containing both the nationally coordinated breeding practices and the nutritional solutions developed to turn immature piglets born in large litters into viable production pigs and high-quality meat. The use of piglets as substitutes for human infants in studies of NEC provided new futures for both pigs and cow colostrum: pigs, originally bred for meat consumption, were turned into near humans in experimental practices; and spray-dried cow colostrum, originally fodder for fragile piglets in industrialized pork production, was potentialized as lifesaving nutrition for preterm infants.

In an interview about the colostrum studies, Professor Per explained to Mie and me: "If one day Biofiber is not here, the colostrum project will end, because I need to have someone to make the irradiation [of the colostrum] and do the testing and so on . . . and to know how to pack the substance and to secure a sterile product [for the clinical studies]." In other words, a long local tradition of turning the substances and lives of pigs and cows into ways to improve human welfare is crucial to the experimental pig studies. Easy access to production pigs, expert knowledge of pig biology, and the low price of production pigs, which researchers often named as the rationale for using the pig as a model organism, grow out of a genealogical connection between life science and agriculture.[20]

When Gunner commented to me that the cow colostrum used for preterm infants had initially been a waste product, I was reminded that the process of translating cow colostrum from farm to clinic is framed as a transformation of waste into value. His comment also opened my eyes to a number of subsequent acts of disposal in substitution practices. In the Newborn Pig Facility, the waste product of cow colostrum is disposed into pig substitutes and absorbed by them, and the substitutes' subsequent disposal (i.e., killing) is crucial to transforming disposable cow colostrum and disposable pigs into nutritional value for infants in the NICU, scientific value for the researchers, and economic value for Gunner's company. In the following section, I turn to the links and separations between cows, pigs, and humans that are part of transforming waste into value.

COLLECTING COW COLOSTRUM AT THE FARM

The role of waste transformer is not new to the Danish pig. In preindustrial farming, Danish pigs lived close to the household and were fed leftovers and other scraps. They literally constituted a garbage bin. They gained their kilos on waste from the farm, and when they reached the right size and Christmas approached, they were killed for the holiday meal, thus releasing their potential for humans.[21] In eating human leftovers and kitchen waste, preindustrial pigs became commensal associates.[22] The Latin word *commensalis* (meaning "sharing a table") is derived from the prefix *com*, meaning "together," and *mensa*, meaning "table" or "meal." As commensal associates, preindustrial pigs became nearly household members (Leach 1964, 51), a kin relationship that was momentarily activated in the researchers' ironic comments about piglets as household members in the lab, as well as in the public outrage about the thousands of piglets that died in industrial barns every day. Furthermore, in experimental practices, the piglets shared a table with calves and human infants by being served a leftover product (cow colostrum) from the same source. Biofiber had a central role in making this commensality possible. For Gunner, the first step toward a shared table was collecting waste.

To make something into waste implies separating a fragment (e.g., cow colostrum) from a whole (e.g., dairy farming).[23] As Catherine Waldby and Robert Mitchell (2006) note in their outline of tissue economies, when tissue is designated as waste, it has been actively detached and cast off from its source. Likewise, by identifying some of the cow colostrum as "surplus" and thus not useful, it is detached from its source, placed in the category of waste, and reevaluated, thus having the potential to enter a new context and substitute for mother's milk in NICUs. The success of this process, as we shall see, depends on the surplus supply of cow colostrum gaining and shedding particular meanings along the way.

On a winter day in 2015, I follow Betina, one of Biofiber's employees, on her visits to some of the dairy farms that deliver colostrum to the company. As one of many tasks that fall under her job title of product supervisor, she makes the initial agreements with the dairy farmers, conducts follow-up visits, and settles accounts between the farmers and the company. In short, she manages all the work that is involved in making farm workers milk the colostrum from cows and carefully move it from the udder to the freezer, where another Biofiber employee collects it to bring to the company's colostrum dairy for quality testing. On this day we are on our way to a new potential contractor. Betina has an appointment with Peter, who supervises the milking of the farm's five hundred cows. Betina parks her van in front of a large redbrick building, one of several buildings that make up this dairy farm in the countryside in southwest Denmark. Betina and I put on white coats and wrap disposable slippers around our boots to avoid letting our invisible passengers of potentially harmful microbes loose in the farm. We follow Peter into the cow yard, where a young Romanian woman passes us with a wheelbarrow. Peter switches from Danish to speak to her in English and then guides us into the area where milking takes place every morning and afternoon.

As Peter takes Betina around the milking area, she inspects the milking equipment used for colostrum collection at the farm. In a humorous, good-natured way, she firmly goes over the procedures, instructing Peter on how to clean the equipment before and after use and how to avoid getting blood, straw, dust, and earwigs in the filled buckets. "We are not interested in suppliers whose quality of colostrum is only good enough for fodder products, but not for human nutrition," she says. Peter and Betina discuss the best location for the freezer so that the milkers will be able to reach it in twenty steps. To make the cow colostrum substitute for the human milk involves sociomaterial processes of washing the milking equipment with soap and water every day; filling buckets (but not to the top, as the liquid increases in size during freezing); taking care that the many other cohabitants at the farm, such as flies and earwigs, do not enter the bucket; and walking straight from the cow to the freezer. For Peter it also involves enrolling specific actors. He explains to Betina that the two Romanian women who work at the farm will be responsible for all of the procedures. In doing so, he reminds me of the important role of migrant workers, who are part of the translational process envisioned to end in the guts of NICU infants in Denmark and China—a global field of interconnected actors I return to in chapter 4.

When Betina inspects the milking equipment, she asks how much colostrum the calves are fed. Peter replies that a newborn calf gets all the colostrum from the first milking. The colostrum yielded from the second milking is what the farm plans to deliver to Biofiber. Shortly afterward, the three of us are seated in the employees' kitchen, talking to the owner of the farm. Over a cup of coffee, he says, "it is good that it [cow colostrum] can be used; otherwise it would be thrown out." At some point in our conversation about the procedures of delivering colostrum to Biofiber, Betina remarks that other farmers who contract with the company include some of the high-quality colostrum from the first milking in the category of "waste" or "surplus colostrum" and therefore receive a higher payment. Betina fully respects the owner's decision to feed his calves all the colostrum from the cow's first milking. "After all, the calves are the ones that secure the farm's future," she says. Nevertheless, her remark elucidates the contingent nature of what makes up both surplus and waste (Svendsen and Koch 2008). This contingency—and its relation to other acts of disposal—comes to the fore in conversations with other farmers who remind me of the routine slaughter of bull calves at birth in conventional dairy production.[24] This disposal practice, which I never witnessed on the farms I visited, may also allow colostrum to dribble into the category of waste.

The porous boundaries around the category of waste hinted at in Betina's conversation with Peter and the owner of the farm were more directly spelled out to me in an interview with Gunner. He explained that as part of Biofiber's ethics policy, the company has explicitly written into its contracts with the farmers that the colostrum delivered to the company is "surplus colostrum" (over-

skudskolostrum), defined as a maximum of two-thirds of the total amount of colostrum per cow. Gunner says: "It is important to us that we are ethically responsible. We do not take the third part meant for the calves." His comment reveals the affective and moral component of substitution, which in this situation comes to the fore when the involved actors take a stance and organize the substitute's relations to its source (production animals) and its new destination (preterm infants). Colostrum from a cow that has newly given birth must secure the survival and health of newborn calves on the farm, but the cow also gains the additional identity of provider of the first milk for preterm infants in NICUs. Gunner tells me that in talking to dairy farmers, he quickly learned that photos of tiny and sick premature infants in the company's newsletter made farmers uncomfortable. Due to the small amounts of colostrum available in the cow's udder compared to dairy milk, collecting colostrum for Biofiber provided the farmers with pocket money, but not a substantial income. Carefully selecting photos of healthy infants for the newsletter, Gunner and his team aimed at maintaining the farmers' engagement. This practice translated cow colostrum from the farm to the clinic by making absent the very infants who would be fed the colostrum.

When the buckets of frozen colostrum are picked up by a Biofiber employee and reach the company's production site, the quality of the frozen colostrum determines its future placement. If a bucket contains impurities (such as blood, earwigs, or flies) or is in other ways contaminated with too many bacteria (every bucket is subjected to thorough testing), the bucket is placed in the corner of a huge freezing area designated for animal fodder for fragile piglets or calves on industrial farms.[25] Making a cow feed infants in the NICU involves not only acts of disposal, but also acts of negotiating the persistent threat of the return of the farm to the clinical setting. When Gunner elaborates on the ethics policy of his company, the policy of "one-third for the calf" is a way of ensuring that the original source of colostrum, nutrition for the calf, does not return in the form of public controversy. When Betina instructs Peter about the hygiene procedures, the processes of washing, cleaning, and walking only twenty steps to the freezer keep traces from the original source (the cow's blood) and its surroundings (flies, earwigs, and straw) at a minimum, so as not to obstruct Biofiber's ability to produce nutrition for humans. When the colostrum's quality is assessed at the company's site, buckets carrying too many traces of the cow and her environment are eliminated, since including them would cause them to reenter the production process in the form of poor inspection reports from the Danish Veterinary and Food Administration. Yet what is filtered out and made absent does not disappear for good (Kevin Hetherington 2004, 162; Svendsen 2011, 427). It may still have some kind of potential agency and cause the farm to reenter settings where it is not wanted. The procedures at the farms and the Biofiber production site illuminate the meticulous work done to establish a viable substitute by creating new

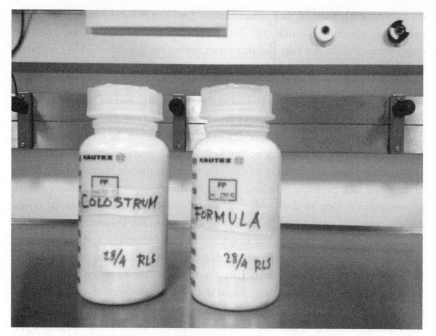

FIGURE 1.1. Cow colostrum and formula to be fed to preterm piglets, Newborn Pig Facility, 2013. Photo by Mie Seest Dam. (Credit: Mie Seest Dam.)

relations and meanings while voiding others. It involves simultaneously fostering kinship between cow and infant through the gut, while keeping the animal at bay. By processing cow colostrum into a dried powder to be reconstituted later in the NICU, the colostrum is further separated from the animal source as part of making it available to human consumers.

FEEDING PIGLETS IN THE ANIMAL FACILITY

Cow colostrum entered the Newborn Pig Facility in a small bucket containing the spray-dried powder, which the team dissolved in water and prepared for feeding the piglets through a syringe. In the fridge, different forms of nutrition (infant formula, human donor milk, and cow colostrum) would be placed next to each other, ready to take out when feeding the piglets every third hour (see figure 1.1). Feeding occupied a central role in the experimental practices. In the standard preterm pig protocols, the piglets were fed intravenously after delivery for two days via an umbilical arterial catheter (parenteral nutrition), a form of feeding that was essential to their survival yet caused intestinal atrophy. Then the piglets were transferred to getting milk directly into their immature gut via a tube (enteral nutrition).[26] This protocol was based on feeding regimes in European NICUs in which infants were also transferred from parenteral to enteral

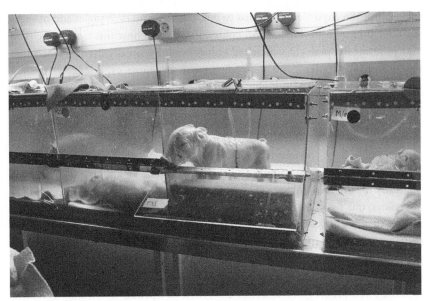

FIGURE 1.2. Preterm piglets in homemade incubator-like boxes before the new facility was built, Newborn Pig Facility, 2011. Photo by the author.

nutrition within the first days of their lives. In the Newborn Pig Facility, the swift transition from parenteral to enteral feeding put the piglets at high risk for developing NEC and thus provided an opportunity to study how the amount of nutrition, the timing of feeding, and the composition of nutrition (cow colostrum, human donor milk, or milk replacers) prevented the disease from becoming severe. Thus, all the activities around the piglets—registering their weight, sex, body temperature; fixing them with catheters; and randomly assigning them to specific groups of enteral nutrition—constituted piglets as substitutes standing in for infants in the experimental setup (what I have referred to as the sociomaterial component of substitution). These activities were meant to ensure that the piglets would become ill from NEC and to study how to reduce adverse effects of the disease. In many respects, preparing food, feeding the piglets, and checking on their condition structured the workday.

During one typical feeding session in 2011, I assisted Swenyu, a graduate student. When I opened the door to the Newborn Pig Facility, the familiar warm, humid air and the cloying odor of feces, milk, and bodies hit me. Along two walls, incubator-like boxes stood next to each other, most of them containing a tiny piglet (see figure 1.2). A litter of about twenty piglets had been delivered by cesarean section a few days earlier, the smallest weighing less than 500 grams. As we approached the incubators, some of the piglets stood on their legs with their eyes open or moved around, while curiously pressing their snouts against the glass or into the mattress. Others were lying down with their eyes closed and looked limp. Swenyu went from box to box, checking on each piglet and observing their bodies, movements, and color. "I don't like how this one looks," she said, pointing out piglet D, which had a blue snout. Eventually she called Morten, one of the veterinarian graduate students who was more experienced than she was, in his office on the floor above and asked him to come down to check the piglet. Although Morten was not on duty according to the schedule, he arrived a few minutes later. Gently touching piglet D's stomach and checking its temperature, he found that its condition was not critical, but he recommended that the team should check the animal every hour. To relieve its visible stomachache, Morten put a tube into its mouth and sucked out some air and mucus.

Ready for the feeding, Swenyu and I marked three syringes with three different colors, one for each of the milk products used in her study, and poured the three different kinds of nutrition into a syringe each. Swenyu then left the three syringes in a bowl with hot water to heat the nutrition and subsequently placed one of the syringes in the bend of her elbow to make sure its contents had reached body temperature. She handed me the syringe with the orange label and took the one with the green label herself. When we opened the incubators whose colors matched that of the syringes in our hands, we noted the amount of milliliters to be fed to the piglet in the box, gently put a hand around it, and poured nutrition into its catheter—keeping an eye on the lines on the syringe to make sure the piglet got exactly the right amount. We alternated between exchanging remarks on the piglets ("Have a look at this one—its hind legs are a bit pale gray, aren't they?") and speaking quietly directly to the piglet ("Hey there, how are you doing?") or communicating to it by making small sounds as if communicating to an infant. At the end of the feeding session we turned each piglet from resting on one side to the other to prevent its lungs from collapsing, a routine that had entered the laboratory after some of the graduate students visited the NICU in Copenhagen and learned the practice. Close to two hours had passed before all piglets had been fed and we switched off the light and closed the door to the piglets' room. In one such situation the week before, the animal technician had ended the feeding session by softly saying, "Goodnight, my babies."

In his ethnographic study of people living with metabolic diseases in India, Harris Solomon (2016) draws on the literal and figurative meanings of "absorption" as a process of both soaking in and being preoccupied, to conceptualize absorption as a dynamic process between body and environment. He argues that absorption is "the possibility for bodies, substances, and environments to mingle, draw attention to each other, and even shift definitional parameters in the process" (5). When the researchers attended to the piglets and carefully let cow colostrum (or other cow-based substances) flow into the pig while keeping a hand around its body, a permeable interface between cow, pig, and human was created. "A mutuality of being" (Sahlins 2011, 2) was conjured up. This way of becoming intrinsic to one another's existence through practices of feeding bears has strong parallels to Carsten's study of relatedness based on fieldwork in Malaysia. There she found that infants sharing milk from the same woman become "milk-siblings" (1995, 227). Her ethnography powerfully reveals that milk kinship is not only bound up with the biological substance of milk but is also crafted by sharing space.

Because we shared space with the piglets and treated them as members of the household, our feeding practices blurred boundaries between bodies and turned the piglets into intimate kin, giving way to a kind of "interspecies milk kinship" (Dam et al. 2017, 130). Substitution relied on letting calf, pig, and infant become commensal associates by eating from the same cow source. These practices crafted interspecies kinship and facilitated translation. Swenyu, with her hands on the piglet and her eyes communicating with it, embodied this process of translation. By mimicking human NICU care in her care for the piglets and feeding them milk substances ultimately meant for human infants, these substitution practices created a space in which pig and researcher were drawn into an intense encounter in which they shared lifesaving (and disease-inducing) substances. In this setting, substitution implied turning piglets into generic proxies, as well as into sentient and intimate kin.

Although Thomas joked about the team's getting "twenty-three children" (see the introduction) and the animal technician addressed the piglets as "my babies," no one in the lab would ever claim that the piglets are human. Their nonhumanness is why they can serve as substitutes and eventually be killed. Yet these humorous remarks reveal opposite meanings that only irony can capture, since irony "entails recognition of being simultaneously both free and determined" (Lambek 2015, 20). The researchers' ironic language suggested to me that they were free to express their intimate relationships with the piglets in the language of kinship but determined to treat the piglets as disposable research tools. The power of the researchers' irony was that it temporarily suspended the boundary between species and made space for uncertainty and ambiguity. However, outside the lab, it became urgent for the researchers to take sides and erect boundaries. This need came to the fore in a seminar discussion about how to enhance the translational value of the pig studies by refining the experimental setup to come closer to the clinical routines in the human NICU. As a response to some of the researchers' suggested way of mimicking the human NICU in the lab setting, one highly esteemed neonatologist who was not directly involved with the study said, "it is important that we are not thinking of the well-being of the pig." With this deliberately provocative comment, he was reminding the group that the otherness of the pig was essential to the strength and potential of their research. Yet the fact that this had to be said points to the power of ambivalence about the pig's identity and reveals "the complexities, paradoxes, and contradictions of . . . experimental animal use" (Sharp 2019, 9), reflecting the affective and moral component of substitution.

Judith Butler writes that "there are deaths that are partially eclipsed and partially marked, and that instability may well activate the frame, making the frame itself unstable" (2016, 75). Might it be that the researchers' discussion of how to improve care for the piglets enacted the animals as partially eclipsed and partially marked, thus exposing, contesting, and destabilizing the frame that turned them into nongrievable creatures? At least the neonatologist felt a need to firmly place the pig in the category of nonpersonal and nonsingular biology, thus reconstituting the frame by maintaining the pig as a generic proxy and, ultimately, a disposable animal. In other words, when piglets were viewed as intimate kin of humans, an equal vulnerability of both human and animal was exposed that brought the "well-being of the pig" to the fore and carried the possibility of seeing it as grievable. This shared vulnerability was crucial to the researchers' efforts to mimic clinical care and turn the piglets into good substitutes, yet at the same time intimate interspecies kinship challenged the dominant notion of piglets as killable and nongrievable.

In his ethnography about the Korowai, a tribal community in West Papua, Indonesia, Rupert Stasch (2009) compellingly demonstrates the central roles of distance, strangeness, and separation in making relations. He argues that the Korowai relate to each other "across margins of combined intimacy and strangeness" (18). I see the researchers, too, as forming relations to the pigs by simultaneously dissolving and remaking boundaries of strangeness.[27] As the conversation about improving clinical care shows, there was no protocol for this moral navigation. While the piglets were by definition (according to both legal framework and cultural consensus) a resource to be used, their use was in itself transformative, potentially threatening the very frame on which the experiment rested. The complex back-and-forth interaction to turn piglets into near humans, all in service of helping translate cow colostrum into the mouths of human babies, illuminated a boundary between human and animal that was in constant flux. In this border zone, the researchers were moral experimenters who allowed piglets to enter the world of the human infant and guided them back again, delineating the sometimes barely discernible boundary between infant and piglet. Forming relations "across [. . .] combined intimacy and strangeness" (Stasch 2009, 18) involved shifting alignments and the painstaking work of sorting out how to combine estrangement and proximity.

FEEDING INFANTS IN THE NICU

During my fieldwork in the NICU in 2010, in the company of a doctor and a nurse, I entered the room of Emily, who had been born two weeks earlier at twenty-five weeks gestation. In contrast to the animal facility, the room contained not twenty-five incubator-like boxes but two well-equipped incubators, each of which was roughly the size of a standard crib. There were two meters between the incubators that contained the unit's smallest infants, Emily being one of them. Close to each incubator was a parent's bed. The NICU sought to facilitate parent-child attachment and had a policy of "family centered care" (Copenhagen University Hospital, 2015).[28] As part of this policy, all parents were encouraged to stay in the NICU as much as possible, sleep next to their child, and be present for the ward round every morning. The NICU also had a family kitchen where parents could prepare small meals and eat at a table. Similar to the way the kitchen in the animal facility constituted a space for taking a break in between attending to the piglets, the family kitchen constituted a space that was separated from the clinical routines, where the parents could rest and exchange experiences.

This morning in Emily's room, her parents sat on their bed next to her incubator. In front of Emily's mother was a mobile stand holding a breast pump. A tube ran from the machine to Emily's mother's breast, which she massaged as the machine pumped. The NICU staff had encouraged Emily's mother to pump out milk as much as possible—preferably every second or third hour in every twenty-four-hour period—so the mobility of the stand was an advantage. Both parents looked anxiously at the three of us in our white coats. The doctor greeted them and said, "We'll take a look at her stomach." Within the first week of her life, Emily had become ill with severe NEC and had had to have an operation. Eight centimeters of her gut had been removed and two ostomy bags put in. On the doctors' rounds the day before, Emily had been described as "very sick, but her situation is stable." This morning there was no imminent danger, but her prospects were uncertain. As a premature infant suffering from NEC, Emily was exactly the kind of infant whose life the pig studies sought to enhance and possibly save.

The doctor attended to Emily in the incubator. She observed Emily's distended stomach, discussed with the nurse the color of the feces in Emily's ostomy bag, and listened to Emily's gut with a stethoscope to detect any gut sounds—which would be a healthy sign. There was no sound. "We hope it [the gut activity] will begin soon. It might take a couple of days," the doctor informed the parents, who attentively followed the inspection. An hour later, I met the father in the hall on his way to put a small container of breast milk in the fridge. At her next meal, Emily was to be fed her mother's milk through a tube. In addition, Emily relied on parenteral nutrition through her bloodstream.

As we saw in the Newborn Pig Facility, the immaturity of the gut complicates digestion, which may cause deadly diseases such as NEC. In particular, the swift transfer from parenteral nutrition to enteral nutrition directly into the gut on day three of the pig studies provokes the disease in the animals and makes it possible to study how different forms of nutrition protect against it. In the NICU, food and fluids are substances without which infants cannot survive, and these fluids are high-risk matters. Which nutrition and extra protein to put in Emily's catheter, what amount, and when to let these substances enter her body are critical

matters to be decided on the daily doctors' rounds. Food is treated like a medication, and feeding exposes both the permeability of body and the environment
and the unpredictability and dangers that lurk at this interface.

When an infant like Emily enters the world prematurely and is brought to the
NICU, all the usual ways in which parents care for their child are suspended. The
mere survival of prematurely born infants is conditional on detaching them from
the bodies of their parents and connecting them to technology and professional
expertise (Landzelius 2003). In these circumstances, attachment between parents and child was difficult. Parents described their infant as looking "alien" or
"animal-like." They feared that the child would not survive and be in their lives
only temporarily, like a guest (Navne, Svendsen, and Gammeltoft, 2018). To
engage parents in the care for their child, staff members taught them how to
tube-feed the child and how to interpret the numbers and sounds produced by
the machines that constantly sustained and monitored the child's health. When
it was medically safe to do so, the infant would be taken out of the incubator and
placed for a while on the naked chest of the mother or father. This practice was
promoted to improve attachment and physical health, and intimate bodily contact between mother and child also introduced the premature child to the breast
and stimulated the mother to produce milk (see figure 1.3). Thus, skin-to-skin
contact was the first step on "The Milky Way" (Copenhagen University Hospital, n.d.)—the title of hospital guidelines on how to attain exclusive breast-
feeding even if the child was born prematurely.[29] The strong focus on parental
involvement reflects a politics of belonging, treating parents and infant as an
inseparable unit and viewing the making of subjects and citizens as highly dependent on the making of families. At the same time, the policies and practices
illustrate how thoroughly the NICU context challenges common ideas about
breast-feeding and family becoming.

Despite the fact that food and feeding practices in the NICU are very far from
either a typical breast-feeding situation or an ordinary meal, the nurses actively
articulated connections between feeding the infant and ordinary food situations.
In referring to individual nutrition schemes listing the diet composition for each
infant, one nurse called these "the menu."[30] The same nurse referred to the dosing cup and the syringe through which the food was provided to the infant as
"knife and fork." In one situation, an infant was relying heavily on parenteral
nutrition through the bloodstream, and the mother's milk was only a supplement. However, after the nurse provided the infant with five milliliters of
mother's milk through a stomach tube, she contentedly remarked, "He has eaten
it all" (*spist op*). In using a language that belongs to just a normal meal for humans
("menu" and "knife and fork") or the ordinary situation of a child eating by itself
("eating it all"), along with emphasizing the importance of mother's milk as the
real meal, these statements and feeding activities morally incorporated the infant
in a family and in human ways of eating. All efforts were put into turning the

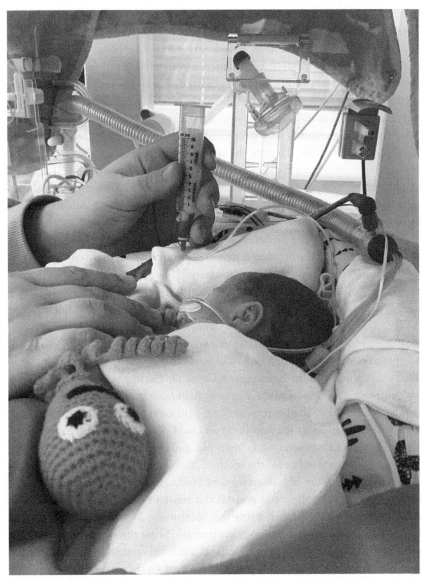

FIGURE 1.3. Mother with child "eating it all," Copenhagen NICU, 2021. Photo by Linda Svenstrup Munk. (Credit: Copenhagen University Hospital.)

alien neonate at the margins of life into a familiar human. Feeding practices attached infants to parents and the human collective.

In interviews in the NICU, parents emphasized that the substance of mother's milk was essential not only to the health and growth of their infant, but also to forming kinship relations.[31] Anders, the father of an infant boy, Mikkel, recounted the first tough days in his son's life. Mikkel, seven weeks old at the time of the interview, had been born by cesarean section at twenty-six weeks gestation. Due to his severe growth retardation, his parents were told that he would probably not survive. Mikkel's mother, Alina, suffered from anemia and preeclampsia and was also in a critical condition. She was admitted to the maternity ward, spending almost three weeks on the floor above the NICU, where her son was receiving vital intensive care. Anders explained that their first days in the hospital had been organized around "a very structured pumping program." Clearly proud of his wife, he elaborated: "Despite the anemia and everything, Alina was able to produce milk even from the very first day. . . . Our schedule would be that Alina would [pump] milk and I would run down [to Mikkel] with even one milliliter." In this setting, not even a tiny drop of milk qualified as waste. Anders further explained that he and his wife ascribed Mikkel's weight gain and his ability to conquer infections to the merits of his mother's milk. As Alina put it, "We know that we've given him the first protection of his whole life." In these conversations, food appeared to be a "pervasive environment" (Landecker 2011, 188) that shaped the biology of the infant's body and crafted parent-child attachment. Thus, following the milky way by pumping, feeding, and absorbing breast milk, Alina, Anders, and Mikkel collaborated as a family to transform Alina's milk into the biology of Mikkel's body and make him become kin.

The intimate work of providing Mikkel with his mother's milk made it possible for Alina and Anders to imagine a future of "healthy survival" and "whole life" for their son. Anders said, "You can't help having a little bit of this feeling that he's the child of the hospital and not your own child . . . and that [feeding him mother's milk] was the first thing we could do." Alina interpreted Mikkel's absorption of what she stressed as "my milk," and the strengths he gained from it, as active acceptance of her as "the mother." Through milky substances and practices and articulations of human ways of feeding, Mikkel's parents conquered their feelings of alienation and reinstated a sense of relatedness between their child and themselves. While it is true that "demonstrating one's humanity entails having corporeal openings out to other beings" (Shaw 2004, 296), in the NICU setting, the openness of premature infants almost threatened their humanness and thus had to be closed in ways that confirmed kinship between parents and child.

COW COLOSTRUM FOR NICU INFANTS

In the Newborn Pig Facility, feeding the fragile piglets and taking care of them became a way to shape them as near humans. In the human NICU, milk actively shaped infants' belonging to the people whose substances they were fed, thus raising concerns among parents about the origin of the substances. Even if mother's milk had first priority, NICU parents were often forced to accept a substitute. When interviewed, they recounted thoughts such as "he [the child] just needs some food," when the nurses asked for their permission to use human donor milk. Nevertheless, relying on food from bodies other than that of the mother raised the questions of, in the words of Solomon, "what it means to be fed by a stranger" (2016, 109) and what relations to craft when feeding "others' milk" (K. Wilson 2018).

Substituting donor milk for mother's milk was connected to feelings of ambivalence. In thinking about the scenario of accepting human donor milk, one mother who had given birth to a boy at twenty-six weeks gestation said: "I would likely become jealous. In particular if he [her child] would gain a relationship to another woman. . . . You pass on something of yourself in the milk."[32] Another mother recounted an incident in which her breast milk had accidentally been fed by a nurse to another child. This made her realize how much feeding her son her own milk meant to her and revealed that breast milk "creates some kind of relation [to the foreign child]," which she experienced as "transgressing." Staff members of the human milk bank located in another hospital shared these concerns. Before initiating a thorough process of pasteurization and quality assessment, they mixed milk from several women to avoid a situation of "my milk to your child," as the bank's director put it. Nevertheless, interviews with the receiving parents illuminated that the milk carried a sticky trace of the connection to the donating woman. It transferred "some imagined relatedness" (K. Wilson 2018, 183), even if only fleetingly. Although many mothers felt that donor milk threatened the exclusive bond between mother and child,[33] their uneasiness was most often a passing feeling and no parents refused to let their child have human donor milk.

When the medical doctor in charge of the randomized controlled pilot study introduced parents to cow colostrum, she presented it as "the first milk," and hence as "designed for newborn babies" in contrast to "mature [human] donor milk" that is "suitable for infants of older age," as it does not contain "all the immunoglobulins and proteins that are important to newborn premature infants." However, a number of parents still emphasized the species origin of the milk and thus perceived mature human donor milk as less alien than cow's milk. These reactions resonate with the experiences of mothers whose children were not introduced to colostrum but who received human donor milk. One of the mothers said, "I didn't have a lot of thoughts about its origin as long as it was from a human being."[34] Another mother noted that human "donor milk is produced for infants. We are the same being (*samme væsen*). We should feed children. Cows provide milk for the calves." Why would NICU parents think of milk from a cow as potentially contaminating, when giving milk to a toddler or drinking it as an adult is usually not considered risky at all?

Along with other parents, Mikkel's father, Anders, reflected upon his own conflicting emotions in relation to cow colostrum: "In the first five seconds it was ugh! . . . Then of course my second reaction was, oh, wait a second, I buy cow's milk every day!" Anders explained that to a person like him who is employed in the pharmaceutical industry, his "professional brain" told him that the spray-dried cow colostrum was "perfectly safe." He concluded that his own reaction was "emotional" and "difficult to explain." It was his wife, Alina, who put words to the bodily reaction of "ugh," which cow colostrum likewise evoked in her: "I see it like this: cow—animal, baby—human. So I think it is also part of nature to be: don't mix those things!" Alina feared that cow colostrum, containing immunoglobulins, would to a greater extent than mature donor milk "take away the mother's chance to provide the baby the first protection"—which would instead originate from a cow.

These conversations reveal the trace effects related to letting cow colostrum substitute for human donor milk. Although cow colostrum was introduced in the clinic exactly because of its positive effects on the immaturity of the infant's gut, it retained traces of an animal substance. The fact that the cow would act as extension of the mother by providing the infant's "first protection" somehow contested the infant's belonging to its parents. Despite the scientific process of fragmenting, separating, and establishing evidence for the positive effect of cow colostrum, for parents there was something difficult to swallow about their infants absorbing it. Cow colostrum had the potential to threaten bodily boundaries and result in an unnatural mix of species. An unwanted mutuality of being with cows and pigs lurked in the wings of these interviews and in some cases became explicit—as in the conversation with Sofie, who jokingly called Amada "our little calf." Another mother explained why she would feel "weird" about feeding cow colostrum to her twins: "It's a bit like if we were having a new heart and then took a heart from a pig. I do think most people would feel weird about that as well, to walk around with a pig's heart, even if it could maybe work." As it appears from these interviews, feeding premature infants with cow colostrum evoked moral ambiguities known from the debate on xenotherapy transplantation of an organ, tissue, or cells between human and pig, a situation that implies not only that a pig is humanized, but also that a "a patient is porcinized" (Sharp 2014, 86). The parents were not troubled by the double animality of the liquid— the way it relied on both cows and pigs—but by the unwelcome continuity or passage between human, cow, and pig. Vinciane Despret suggests that we view the transplantation of cells or organs from one being to another as an instance of metamorphosis, in which the transformation of bodies involves a transformation of beings (2016, 190). I believe that the "weirdness" reflects the parents' shivering at such an unpredictable and multidirectional transformation. Interspecies kinship was crafted in a way that put the child in close engagement with beings from which it should be separated, thus questioning the child's humanness and potentially separating the child from its human parents.

Amanda's pet name of "our little calf" is premised on the fact that no parent seriously thought that feeding an infant cow colostrum would turn it into a calf. The parents who agreed to be part of the randomized controlled pilot study and to give cow colostrum as a supplement to their infant did so because they considered cow colostrum the best alternative to mother's milk. Nevertheless, the yuck factor remained. In the NICU, the animal origin of cow colostrum and research piglets implied something dangerous that threatened the infant's attachment not only to its parents, but also to the human collective. By repetitively reifying and reaffirming the preterm infant as human, the responses of the parents illuminated exactly how premature infants are near human and flexible species like the research piglets. The NICU infant at the edge of life was also at the edge of humanity. Species and kinship belonging were precarious in the NICU, and both the substance fed to the child and the practice of feeding were ways of including the child in the category of the human. By staying with a human milk diet, the parents guarded the humanness of their child and reclaimed themselves as parents.

In the animal facility, this interspecies milk kinship was crucial to translating cow colostrum from the farm to the clinic. In the NICU, interspecies kinship did not facilitate translation, but hindered it. The animal origin of the colostrum reduced the acceptability of translating the positive results in the pig studies into clinical studies on human infants. What cut across the Newborn Pig Facility and human NICU was that the species flexibility of both piglets and infants provoked strong boundary-policing responses. To the medical doctor in charge of the clinical study in Copenhagen, the interviews with the parents made it evident that more information about the biogenetic relatedness between calf, piglet, and infant would not necessarily make the parents more willing to let their child participate in the cow colostrum study. She decided to stress the good evidence for using cow colostrum but leave out details about the cows and the pig studies. It was by becoming the invisible transformer of cow colostrum into infant nutrition that the pigs in the studies successfully carried cow colostrum from the dairy farms to the NICU.

MAKING COW COLOSTRUM BIOAVAILABLE

On the last day of the NEOMUNE seminar in 2014 at the seaside hotel outside Copenhagen, I talked to Annette, one of Biofiber's employees. She was closely involved in making the company's colostrum product live up to legislation and quality controls for human nutrition and in designing the small, handy ten-gram packages of spray-dried colostrum suitable for meal portions in the clinic. Excitedly, Annette described to me the day when the first infant was included in the randomized pilot study in the Danish NICU and fed Biofiber's colostrum product: "We watched the phone constantly. If they called from the clinic and told us that the infant had thrown up, we would have to close down that whole production." With relief, Annette told me that the infant did not throw up: the colostrum product was not haunted by traces of the farm, and it did not return to waste. Cow colostrum had been successfully carried across from the cow, through the pigs, to a child. The translation was complete.

Annette's anxiety, communicated concurrently with her enthusiasm for the colostrum product for human infants, concerned the bioavailability of the product. In pharmacology, bioavailability is a well-known concept that refers to the degree to which a substance can be used by the parts of the body on which it is intended to have an effect. The first time an infant body was given cow colostrum—followed by numerous infants in both China and Denmark between 2013 and 2018—proved that the colostrum had a high degree of bioavailability. If we follow Aditya Bharadwaj (2008) in letting the concept of bioavailability refer also to the geopolitical, moral, and social processes through which a body becomes ready to enter specific scientific or clinical practices, we can see that the reproductive and geopolitical history of breeding and producing pigs in Denmark has been central to shaping the pig as an available and ethically unproblematic resource and as kin. Next, making the cow colostrum substitute for human milk and piglets substitute for human infants implies treating calves, piglets, and infants as being of the same kind and letting them eat from the same source. Substitution unsettles species borders and facilitates interspecies milk kinship. In the Newborn Pig Facility, interspecies milk kinship is essential to producing data, which in the form of scientific evidence can travel into the clinic. The whole process of bioavailability relies on crafting a mutuality of being among cows, pigs, and human, yet at the very last step when introducing cow colostrum—bolstered by scientific evidence—the involved researchers and clinicians realize that for parents to accept the absorption of this liquid gold, the mutuality of being needs to be made invisible. For cow colostrum to flow into infant bodies in a friction-free way, a moral landscape of separate kinds and firm species boundaries was essential. Relatedness in the form of biological connection (pigs as generic proxies) and intimacy (pigs as intimate kin) grounded the whole translational endeavor, yet in the end it challenged "the most powerful and enduring of cultural constructions of kinship relations, that between mother and child" (Hird 2004, 227).

Acts of disposal are central to realizing substitution and converting agricultural waste—via disposable pig bodies—into life-giving substances for the reproduction of human society (healthy infants). However, when we step closer to these processes of replacement, what comes to the fore is the anxiety about interspecies kinship they provoked and the fear of "kinship's betrayal through shared substance" (Solomon 2016, 119).[35] In the context of human-animal relationships in villages in Central Himalaya, Govindrajan argues that "multispecies relatedness draws as much on incommensurable difference as ineffable affinity" (2018, 4). Likewise, creating bioavailability by connecting cow, pig, and infant through colostrum relied as much on dissolving species boundaries as on forging them. In the end, delegating the near human piglet to biological life (as the neonatologist did in the seminar) and making the colostrum testing process invisible (as was necessary in the clinic) become effective ways of recognizing the human and situating this human in intraspecies kinship. For the people engaged in this work, substituting piglets for infants and cow's colostrum for human donor milk demanded skills and work far beyond the biological modeling of the pig. It involved continuous processes of forging interspecies kinship and erasing it to create a substitutive arrangement in which the cow acted as an extension of the mother by lending her colostrum without threatening the human mother as original. Making cow colostrum bioavailable illuminates the human in the animal and the animal in the human, but this porosity also provoked border and maintenance practices. To parents, it became important to guard the humanness of fragile infants and build their selves as human through intraspecies kinship.

I take these insights into kinship as my point of departure for the next chapter, which explores how practices of care and killing are at the core of substitution. Not only are borders between species made and erased in making the pig substitute for the human, but so are borders between life and death. As the next chapter shows, laboratory practices of caring for piglets at the margins of life, killing them at the end of the experiment, and turning them into tissue samples reveal new layers of the moral complexity of substitution.

2 · KILLING
Pigs as Sacrificeable Beings

"I always begin with the infants. If people think it sounds interesting, I'll go on and say I work with nutrition . . . and then tell them that I work with a pig model to investigate disease in infants," Marie, a postdoctoral researcher, says. She is answering my question about how she presents her work to strangers. I am interviewing three researchers from the Newborn Pig Facility, and Lone, a graduate student, supports Marie's view: "You cannot touch a premature infant [for research]. Everyone agrees that you are not allowed to work with (*pille ved*) a sick premature infant at the margins of life. That's why we use the pig."

In this conversation, the pig enters the scene as a substitute for a human infant, who is precious and urgently needs a cure but cannot be experimented on. Nutritional supplements, like the cow colostrum used by NEOMUNE, must be demonstrated to be safe in nonhuman models before it can be used in human trials. Sufficiently similar in terms of biology, but morally different, the pig steps in and substitutes for the child. As Marie's stepwise presentation of her research to strangers reveals, this substitution is not without moral implications. To avoid negative reactions from their listeners, Marie and Lone are careful to place animal experimentation within the larger moral project of saving infants' lives. For Marie, this larger project was not only a strategic presentation of her research. As she noted in another conversation, "to me it makes a huge difference that I work with animals for the sake of the clinic. I can't say that I will never work for the cosmetics industry, but I would definitely have great difficulty working with animals for cosmetics." Her comment hints at the affective struggles related to attending to sick piglets, killing them, turning them into samples, and being accountable to the public.

The exchange envisioned—pig lives for human lives—epitomizes the pig as a generic but valuable life, open to a particular kind of exchange. Being outside the moral collective of humans, the animal's life is calculated as less worthy than the human's life, and precisely for this reason it is possible to treat the animal as a substitutive research subject (C. Thompson 2013) that is not merely disposable, but sacrificeable. When animals substitute for human subjects, the violence that is part of experimental biomedicine—and that prior to the implementation of the Nuremberg Code was also practiced on some groups of humans—is transferred to the animal. Put differently, the researchers' framing of their work tells a classic salvation story: the animal's suffering promises to relieve human suffering.[1] As Michael Lynch (1988) has pointed out, laboratory life consecrates the animal and transforms it from a naturalistic animal into an analytical entity that has the potential of producing scientific breakthroughs.

Legislation on the use of animals in science reflects this moral economy. A directive from the European Union (EU) simultaneously positions the animal as holding "intrinsic value which must be respected" (2010, paragraph 12) and legitimizes the killing of the animal for a higher purpose. The Danish guidelines, which build on EU legislation, state that a "considerable benefit" (*væsentlig gavn*) for humans, animals, or plants should be expected before an animal experiment can be approved (Danish Ministry of Food and Agriculture 2014, section 8). When a nonhuman animal is doing work for a species—improving the health of its own or the human species—killing is no longer considered a routinized act as in the slaughterhouse but gains the character of a sacrifice. This sacrificial logic also has a linguistic presence in the field of animal-based experimental science, where "sacrifice" is a normal term for the acts that lead to the death of an animal in an experiment.

Despite the centrality of sacrifice in the Newborn Pig Facility—as trope and as technical term—many of the researchers I followed disliked the term when directly asked about it. When referring to the killing of animals in science, they called it "euthanizing" (*eutanasi*) or "putting down" (*aflivning*). Among themselves in daily interactions in the laboratory, they would also say "kill" (*slå ihjel*) and refer to the last day of the study as "kill day" or "dissection day." Although these terms have very different meanings (I return to this point below), none of them bear the religious connotations of sacrifice. To the researchers, caring for a piglet and killing it at the end of a study was part of their job. That work was a requirement of graduate or postgraduate studies of gut development, microbiota, and human nutrition, as well as a stepping-stone to jobs in agribusiness, the pharmaceutical industry, and academia. They saw their work as related to basic scientific and applied questions. Nevertheless, laboratory duties with the piglets made up a major part of their scientific work, and this work was rooted in the envisioned exchange of pig lives for human lives, which inescapably contained the logic of sacrifice.

APPROACHING LIFE, SUFFERING, AND DEATH IN EXPERIMENTAL PRACTICES

How is it possible to treat pigs as near human and maintain them as sacrificial animals? What is the role of death in interspecies kinship? In this chapter, I answer these questions by ethnographically entering the sacrificial exchange while at the same time taking seriously the fact that researchers in their daily laboratory routines do not see their work with piglets as consisting of extraordinary events. Consequently, I do not conceptualize the experimental work as a ritual or religious process, instead exploring the practices of turning piglets into human substitutes in ordinary laboratory routines. In doing this, I take inspiration from Lesley Sharp's fascinating book on moral negotiations among personnel in animal laboratories (2019). In uncovering the moral dimensions of suffering and death in the laboratory, Sharp encourages her readers to think beyond the trope of sacrifice, as this term so easily positions the animal as a gift to science rather than as a subject and work partner. Like Sharp, I am interested in the intimate world of human-animal relationships in experimental practices, and thus I follow her recommendation to investigate these moral complexities in everyday work practices. However, rather than discarding sacrifice as a conceptual framework, I wish to enrich the framework of sacrifice by bringing the scholarly work on sacrifice as an exchange of life into conversation with multispecies ethnography.

One might imagine that taking care of very sick piglets and then turning them into biological samples is an emotionally challenging experience. This was not the case. During my first weeks in the Newborn Pig Facility, using pigs as a research tool was continuously presented as closely connected to, and almost a natural extension of, Danes' long history of treating the pig as a resource. The researchers often expressed the sentiment that, as one of them put it, "as a nation we have decided to produce pigs for food, and the small numbers we use here are nothing compared to the pork production. The piglets in here have much better lives than the ones in industrialized farming." I would follow up by positioning myself as a pork-eating Dane and mention that both of my parents grew up on farms. In addition, I spent my childhood summer vacations on my father's parents' small farm, which included a pigsty. These "animal use positions" (C. Thompson 2013, 210) instilled self-evidence into routines of removing dirt from pig bodies, weighing them, estimating their suffering and relieving their pain, mixing their milk diet, feeding them, and in the end cutting them up and turning them into samples. The agribiopolitics, which came to the fore in these routines, treats the governing of the wealth and health of the national population as intertwined with the governing of pig lives, based on a dividing line between human and pig. This dividing line resonated with the human exceptionalism that undergirded the material practices of maintaining pigs in industrialized barns and eating pork as a daily food. The moral ordering of relations between sovereign (human) subjects and an exploitable (pig) resource made the practices of letting live and letting die seem unremarkable.

At the School of Veterinary Medicine and Animal Science, where the Newborn Pig Facility was located, agribiopolitics was not only an abstract arrangement of enabling the human population to thrive by making livestock thrive.

Agribiopolitics was also materially present. As I entered the campus on my bike, I passed the beautiful garden of the school, which had been built in 1860 in the Romantic style of the period. Right next to the garden was the house where all cadavers used in teaching and research were stored before being sent off for disposal. Sometimes an acrid stench hung in the air. At other times, there was a more pleasant smell of stables, coming from the surrounding buildings that housed livestock. Just around the next corner, I arrived at the ordinary looking mid-twentieth-century yellow brick building that contained the Newborn Pig Facility. During my first period of fieldwork, the door to the building was open during the day, and I could walk directly into the facility. To me, the open door reflected the obviousness of the animal-use position in the setting and the absence of threats from animal rights activists. Yet there was no sign on the door signaling to the outsider what the building contained, an absence that expressed an awareness that the animal-use position might not be shared by everyone. Some years later, a new university policy of locked doors at all campuses was introduced, and I had to ring a bell to be admitted.

Inside the yellow brick building, animal use was omnipresent. In the first study I followed, I would often meet Rikke, an animal technician, who went from box to box checking the condition of each of the piglets, and Lone, a graduate student, who prepared the milk for the piglets in the small room next door. In following these routines, my field notes expressed a great deal of disorientation. What should I write down about the clinical assessment of the piglets and the administration of the nutrition practices, which appeared so undramatic? How could I compose a meaningful anthropological story about trivial conversations and interactions among researchers, animal technicians, and piglets in incubators? Even death and dissection became routine. More than once, I found myself longing to return to my earlier fieldwork in clinical genetics clinics and in vitro fertilization clinics, where on a daily basis I had witnessed moving conversations about beginnings and endings of life. Yet as my fieldwork progressed—especially as I began interviewing members of the team—I was alerted to the researchers' and animal technicians' affective responses to witnessing the suffering and death of piglets so intimately. For the people working in the Newborn Pig Facility, attending to piglets in incubators was, on the one hand, a common part of their everyday work in nutritional science. On the other hand, these ordinary routines were about administering and taking responsibility for piglet lives that were highly unstable and continuously involved extraordinary moments of care and life-and-death decision making. If in one moment I embraced the straightforwardness and normalness of animal use, in the next moment the researchers' skilled and careful handling of the small pig bodies reminded me of the imbrication of the morally extraordinary in the ordinary, revealing the tactile and affective dimensions of substitution.

Daily experimental practices spelled out to me that (the hope of) extending the lives of humans is paradoxically enabled via the loss of lives. Running experiments involved acts of unmaking the world (imposing suffering and death on piglets) as part of making the world (enhancing science and contributing to welfare and health for humans).[2] In this chapter, I describe how the researchers interact with the piglets in these processes. I see the experimental space as "an enabling structure" (Lien 2015, 126) that allows piglets to appear as both biological and biographical lives. I pay close attention to how configurations of life as biology and biography are related to practices that make piglets appear as sentient and nonsentient beings. I track how during the course of the experiment, pigs are established first as nonsentient biological life, then momentarily and fleetingly as grievable individuals with a biography, and finally as killable research subjects. Killing the pig is crucial to the completion of the intimate kin relationship with the pig, as this act holds the promise of future health for human infants. I then discuss sacrificeability by considering the process through which the last nonhuman primates in Danish laboratories—in contrast to the pigs—have moved out of this category.

GETTING THE PIGLETS UP AND RUNNING

"You can be certain that there will be many holes to sew," the professor enthusiastically told her students as she cut through the stomach of the pregnant sow and ripped off some fatty tissue. A splash sounded as the blood hit the floor. It was a Monday morning in November 2009, and we were in the middle of another cesarean section, marking the beginning of a new study in the laboratory. The research team was gathered around the sow, ready to receive the piglets and transfer them to incubators in the room next door. For the next five days, the team would take turns caring for the piglets both day and night. Standing in front of the anesthetized pregnant sow, who weighed 250–300 kilos and was lying silently with her tongue hanging out of her mouth, the professor's comment about "the many holes to sew" hinted at the stitching skills she wanted her students to practice before the sow was killed later in the day. The professor then lifted one piglet after another out of the womb. At a sign from the professor, Lone injected a needle into what to me looked like a bubble or balloon in the uterus, and with the needle she extracted the amniotic fluid. Some of it contained blood, and Lone discarded that immediately, allowing only the clear fluid from the needle to be transferred to plastic containers.

The performance of the cesarean section—with the huge body in the middle of the room surrounded by a crowd of people talking about its size and making guesses about the number of piglets in its womb—made the sow appear as a nonsentient vessel from which educational experience, piglets, and amniotic fluid could be harvested. Similarly, the still anesthetized piglets brought to the incubator room and enrolled in the laboratory space appeared as nonsentient material to which catheters and feeding tubes were attached. Checking on the well-being of a piglet, Rikke commented on its size and pink color and said, "He's a million"—referring to the piglet's potential for thriving within the experimental setup and providing good data. Looking at another one, which was bleeding from the umbilical cord, she said, "Oh, what is happening here?" She then took action to stop the bleeding. In a similar situation in another experimental week, I noticed that Rikke left the most precarious piglets, which were often the ones weighing less than 500 grams, as the last ones to be given a letter (by which the piglets were known) on the Excel spreadsheets. She did this so the piglets could more easily be deleted from the cohort if, as expected, they could not be made viable. As I interpreted these situations, low birth weight or very superficial breathing represented an undesirable specificity and individuality, illustrating that the aim of this initial phase of the experiment was not simply to make the piglets survive as individuals but to create a workable experimental system. The valuation and selection of pig lives implied measuring the piglets' potential for providing good data and in the end contributing to robust scientific results, public health, agribusiness, and future funding. In other words, the value of the piglet in the experiment was questioned only when doubts were raised about its ability to become part of knowledge infrastructures and translational efforts.

In these first hours after the cesarean section, a frequent question among the researchers when checking the piglets was, "is it up and running?" (*er der gang i den?*). By "up and running," they referred to the accomplishment of making "it"—the newborn piglet—viable within the experimental system. This involved making it breathe by swinging it in a tea towel or massaging its body, keeping it warm in the incubator, measuring its weight and well-being, identifying its sex, inserting catheters to connect its body to the feeding machine, providing it with a letter, allocating it to a treatment group, and registering it all in Excel spreadsheets in the computer. "Up and running" metaphorically represented the pig body as a machine to be started, and it also pointed to the close connection between starting a pig life and establishing the experiment—despite the fact that the piglets were parts in, rather than the entirety of, the experimental system. If it is true that metaphors provide a core image around which moral understandings of the good are proposed (Mattingly 2014, 158), the researchers' use of the machine metaphor signals that for them, the highest good is seeing and treating breathing pig bodies as the crux of generating knowledge about nutrition and gut maturation.

The senior people in the laboratory also sometimes articulated their work as "running the machine." This term referred not only to doing work on the piglets, but also to applying for research funding, entering into collaborative relationships with nutrition companies and international scientists, giving lectures, enrolling graduate students in the laboratory, supervising students, and turning samples into scientific papers and PhD dissertations. Although these activities went beyond the space of the Newborn Pig Facility, they all had a connection to the skilled work of getting the piglets "up and running," thus creating an experimental system. The piglet bodies in the experiments were at the heart of the scientists' collaborations with clinical and industrial partners, their educational commitments and responsibilities, and their research production.

The work on the piglets' bodies—which often consisted of a senior scholar instructing a junior scholar while the radio played something soft and other colleagues were chatting casually—always reminded me of the atmosphere in Danish bicycle repair shops. The pigs were treated as disarticulated parts, with experienced hands putting feeding tubes through the mouth into the stomach and inserting catheters into an artery in the umbilical cord. "Anyone can insert a catheter," Thomas told me when I witnessed this work on my first day of fieldwork in 2009, thus underlining the routinized aspect of catheter insertion and its undramatic character (see figure 2.1). While using needle and thread to stitch feeding tubes and catheters to the cheeks and abdomens of the still anesthetized piglets, the researchers discussed the national television news from the previous night, commented on the poor respiration of a piglet they did not expect to live through the next hours, or exchanged humorous comments about the swine flu—caused by the H1N1 influenza virus—which was then entering Denmark. On leaving the laboratory after such days of cesarean section and placing the piglets in their boxes, I had the confusing feeling that no existential issues had been at stake. Tiny piglets were born with pulses that made their bodies move up and down. Nonetheless, what happened appeared not as issues of life and death, but rather as a question of instrumentalizing biological life by connecting the piglets to other laboratory players and simultaneously detaching the animals from their species (the sow).

On this first day of the study, the laboratory processes appropriated the pigs, transforming them into nonsentient surfaces on which the experiment as a tool carved out a substitute for the human as part of educating a new generation of scholars, contributing to science, and sustaining human health and wealth. "Up and running" implied a successful configuration of pig bodies as nonsentient biological life, which through emplacement in the laboratory could be turned into the raw material of science. The machine metaphor captured the sociomaterial aspects of substitution, making the pig gain nearness to the human in terms of biology and treatment while remaining, as my friend insisted "just a pig" (see prologue).

CARING FOR PIGLETS

Within the first twenty-four hours after the cesarean section, as the piglets woke up from the anesthesia, they gradually gained individuality. Their eyes opened, and some of them stood up and bumped around in their incubators, sniffing

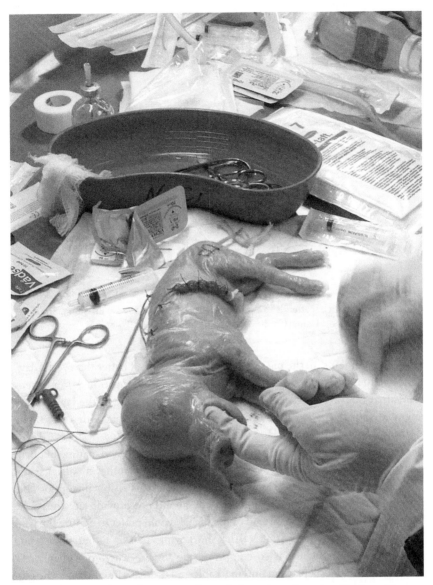

FIGURE 2.1. An anesthetized preterm piglet ready for catheter insertion, Newborn Pig Facility, 2013. Photo by Mie Seest Dam. (Credit: Mie Seest Dam.)

curiously. Others remained lying down and looked pale. During the first two days, one or two people were always on watch over the piglets both day and night. Born prematurely, the piglets were extraordinarily precarious lives and were fully dependent on human care to stay alive.[3] A log book was kept on each piglet, in which the researcher on watch registered quantifiable numbers for food intake and weight, listed individual treatments such as oxygen and painkillers, and

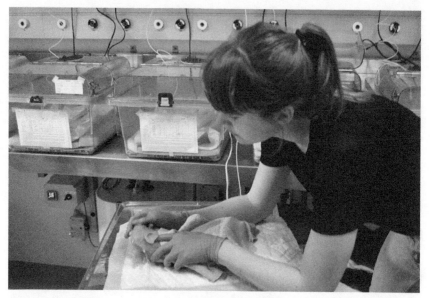

FIGURE 2.2. A researcher attends to a preterm piglet, Newborn Pig Facility, 2013. The researcher is Mie Seest Dam. (Credit: Mie Seest Dam.)

included comments on the pig's situation (e.g., "weak but better than yesterday," "sensitive to noise," or "lying on the side, but reacts to stimulation"). For experiments that ran several weeks, this record of the piglet's life in the lab came to resemble a medical record for a patient and provided the pig with a biography (Dam and Svendsen 2018, 359).

One day, Rikke attended to a piglet that was not thriving and, patting her own stomach, said, "its stomachache sure must be painful." In another situation, when Thomas was putting a catheter in a piglet, the animal was visibly uncomfortable with the intervention. Explaining to me why he did not provide anesthesia, he said, "if it was me [suffering instead of the pig], I would prefer to endure the pain [related to inserting the catheter] the short while it lasts rather than going through anesthesia, which is so compromising for the whole body." In these exchanges, which took place in unremarkable and ordinary interactions, the piglets were not unspecified nonsentient life merely reacting to microbiota. They were sentient lives placed in relationship to the researchers who fed them individually, changed their diapers, identified with them, and made great efforts to reduce the pain they might experience (see figure 2.2). Rikke's and Thomas's comparisons between the piglets' bodies and their own human bodies testify to the way "the body is . . . unbound" (Butler 2016, 52), which made the humans in the room experience precariousness as a condition shared by humans and pigs.

The experiment forced the absorption of the nutrition products and existence in the human-controlled environment on the piglets at the same time as these laboratory routines facilitated the incorporation of the piglets into the researchers' lives. One day in 2011 when feeding the piglets, Swenyu and Morten, two graduate students, talked about the intense work of attending to the animals 24/7 through an experimental week. Swenyu remarked that during her first experience of caring for research piglets, she would have liked to have had her bed moved into the piglets' room. Morten laughed and agreed with her. He recalled his first night watch in the lab, during which he got no sleep as he was so attentive to the fragile piglets and constantly ready to intervene. In addition, the unfamiliar noise from the feeding machines made him worry that they were not functioning properly. Swenyu's comment was ironic, as she was not seriously considering putting a bed in the piglets' room. Yet as chapter 1 showed, ironic comments convey opposite meanings. In this case, the students' comments treated the piglets as biological expendable lives and simultaneously as biographical lives in a close relationship to the researchers. The researchers' absorption in the lives of the piglets made them take in the unpredictability of the animals' urgent situation. Joking about sleeping next to the piglets like a parent illuminates the permeable boundaries between researcher, piglet, and the laboratory environment in producing good data. As Thomas explained to Mie Seest Dam, one of my graduate students, and me, "[You need] to be conscious of the pain of the animal. . . . Your own feeling for the animal has to tell you if the pain is weak or strong. . . . How would you feel if your condition was like that [of the pig]?"[4]

In asking these questions, an absolute moral difference between human and animal dissolves. The piglet's capacity to suffer establishes "a relation of touching and being touched, a relation of responsiveness and responsibility" (Bruns 2011, 84). In putting himself in the place of the piglet, Thomas expressed a multi-directionality and openness in his exchange with the animals. This mutuality involves a "capacity to 'read' the other, to register and respond to each other's presence" (Clark 2007, 62). He stepped into the space of the piglet and included the pig in the community of humans (not the reverse). Marie, who was a graduate student in my first period of fieldwork and in the following years worked in the lab as a postdoctoral student, described the way she engaged with the suffering piglets by populating the place with the animals:

It [estimating the piglet's suffering] is very subjective. I may have a feeling of how conscious the piglet is, because I often feel that when they have NEC [necrotizing enterocolitis] it is as if they become distant—it's the way I feel it myself, and it may be wrong, that if one could measure its pain it would turn out to be in intense pain. . . . In other situations, it is as if they are stressed or suffer in other ways. Once, in connection with a caesarean, which had taken a long time, I found that several pigs were in poor shape, you know, were restless, limping and whined a bit. I felt very bad about it because it seemed that they were aware of the fact that they were in pain.[5]

With no definitive method by which she could measure the pain of the piglets, Marie attended to them as animals with whom she shared the condition of mortality, suffering, and the capacity of having a point of view. Here, Talal Asad's outline of the relationship between suffering and agency captures what is at stake: "Addressing another's pain is not merely a matter of judging referential statements. It is about how a particular kind of moral relationship can be inhabited and enacted" (2000, 42). We may understand the kind of moral relationship that Marie described as a process of compassionately "being alongside" (Friese 2019, 295; Latimer 2013). She attached to the piglet by stepping into its position and acting as an extension of it based on her own corporeal experience. Yet she preserved her own perspective ("it's the way I feel it myself, and it may be wrong"), thus remaining distinctly human. This "relational extension," as Joanna Latimer calls it, "preserves a sense of difference at the same time as it performs partial connectedness and mutuality" (2013, 99). I see this "relational extension" as central to the researchers' practice of substitution. In the case of Marie and the piglet, substitution does not only signify the identity of the piglets as substitutes for infants by carrying their disease. Substitution is also a condition for the work of the researchers, who substitute for the animal by partially inhabiting the position of the piglet and acting as an extension of it ("How would you feel if your condition was like that [of the pig]?") and being open to carrying its condition and well-being.[6]

When treating piglets in pain, the researchers had to make difficult decisions. On the one hand, euthanization may sometimes seem the most benevolent approach toward the individual suffering piglet. On the other hand, the researchers needed statistically significant results and hence needed a certain number of piglets to survive through the last day of the study. If too many piglets are euthanized early, a whole new litter may need to be enrolled in the experiment, thereby compromising the ethical principle of using as few animals as possible in a given research project.[7] As I heard numerous times in conversations among the researchers, "a euthanized piglet costs a piglet at the other end" (*det koster en gris i den anden ende*). "The other end" refers to the monetary costs of enrolling one more litter in the experiment, the laborious and time-consuming work of running the study, and the suffering of these future piglets that substitute for the euthanized ones. Thus, "the other end" points to the landscape of "running the machine," which puts pressure on the researchers to reach scientific results, stick to project plans, and complete doctoral studies within timeframes established by grant proposals. In treating suffering piglets, the researchers were painfully aware of two needs: to act benevolently toward the individual pig and to gather good data and thereby make all the laboratory work and piglet suffering worth the trouble. Rikke, who was responsible for the daily handling of the piglets, described it this way:

We have this debate—and have had it since we started this experiment: how far should we go when these piglets get sick. The point is that if we kill them early we won't get significant results, and it's useless and the life of the piglet is wasted, and that is sad. But I also feel uncomfortable when we have prolonged the process and realize that the piglets suffer, that they are afraid and in pain . . . you see the fear in their eyes and in such situations I just feel they have to be put down, I just can't stand it.[8]

In these deliberations about balancing what is good for science with what is good for the piglet, Rikke starts out by presenting the moral economy of the experimental practice—namely, that the experiment is a tool with which to create human health. From this perspective, a piglet that is killed before it becomes seriously ill is a "waste" of potential, as the team will lack "significant results." Yet while talking about the pain of the piglets, Rikke talks just as much about her own moral malaise as about the animals' pain. She describes being emotionally moved by the piglets and engages in a form of corporeal exchange in which existential affinity for a moment removes the notion of the piglet as simply raw material for science. As we saw in the case of Marie, being moved emotionally creates a moral relationship across the species divide, and in Rikke's case, her sense of morality contests the ethical principle of reduction (i.e., avoiding having to enroll another pig in the experiment). In this situation, to act morally becomes equivalent with ending the suffering of the piglet by putting it down. Yet Rikke's intimacy with the piglet does not mean that she becomes a whole with the pig. She does not enter a totalizing togetherness with the piglet. Rather, Rikke has her own concerns that differ from those of the pig, as she will be the one to decide "how far to go," as she puts it. In Rikke's description, substitution encompasses both the sociomaterial practice of turning pigs into substitutes suffering from the same disease as preterm infants and the intimacy of stepping into the piglet's position and partially inhabiting its world.

It would be a mistake to understand the care for sentient individual piglets as running counter to the experiment as an experimental system, in which piglets are turned into research tools. As the researchers told me many times, continuous attention to the condition of individual piglets is crucial to collecting good data. Individual care is part of making piglets viable within the study and "running the machine." During my years in the Newborn Pig Facility, the researchers' collaboration with clinicians from the NICU increased the individual care that had already been present in the lab. In some experimental settings, efforts to improve care in animal research (e.g., by environmental enrichment) may run counter to the scientific ideal of controlling the environment and thus hinder translation to a clinical setting (see Nelson 2018). In contrast, in the Newborn Pig Facility, the researchers and clinicians saw individual care as a way to model a clinical situation, thus enhancing the reliability of their data and their possibilities for translation. As Carrie Friese (2013b) has shown in her pioneering study of care in laboratory practices, care plays a constitutive role in the organization of the experimental practice, shaping the animal bodies and the findings that result from them. In the Newborn Pig Facility, there was continuous discussion about which forms of individual care to incorporate into daily laboratory practices and which to leave out. In these negotiations, the standardization aimed for in the experiment had to be balanced with the care needed to keep piglets alive.[9]

MORAL PERILS

In her study of using actors as substitutes for patients in U.S. medical schools, Janelle Taylor demonstrates that substitution "reconciles . . . the moral commitment to avoid suffering with the . . . commitment to realistically portray it" (Taylor 2011, 159). This was exactly what researchers in the Newborn Pig Facility faced. In a group discussion that Mie and I set up with researchers in June 2013, Marie asked: "The pig is a valuable resource. We don't want it to die [before the scheduled time]. But [on the other hand] our individual treatment may also prolong suffering. So what are the ethics here?"[10] In asking this question, Marie did not refer to animal ethics as understood within a bioethical framework of institutionalized rules and guidelines of professional conduct. In all their practices, the researchers carefully followed bioethical codes of conduct. Instead, Marie alluded to the ways in which the "ethics" of realistically producing and portraying the suffering of infants in pig substitutes always had to be lived through one's own body and sensations and was situated in specific spaces and unique interactions ("here"). In other words, she hinted at the moral peril (Mattingly 2014, 15) that each study holds.

Such moral peril increased during studies in 2013, which investigated how nutrition affects brain development. In these studies, the pigs were divided into groups according to what they were fed (milk formula, cow colostrum, or human donor milk). The pigs' cognitive development was tested across twenty-six days by carrying out behavioral tests as well as EEG (a method to record brain electrical activity) and MRI (an image analysis system to record volumes and activities in brain regions). The behavioral tests involved making the piglets navigate a maze to obtain a milk reward (see Andersen et al. 2016). Since the standard preterm model ran for five days, it was a huge expansion to let the sometimes severely compromised piglets live for more than twenty days in the laboratory. Only intensive care and individual treatment made it possible for these highly compromised piglets to remain alive to the last day of the study and produce good data, thus paving the way for the next research phase of analyzing samples, writing papers, and presenting results for pediatricians. Yet continuous treat-

ment also meant "prolonged suffering," as Marie phrased it. In the case of euthanasia before the scheduled time, the piglet would be relieved of its suffering, but
it would not provide good data, and its life as a "valuable resource" would be
wasted. While Marie "doesn't want it to die," as she said, taking care of the precarious piglets also involved affective struggles.

On a Friday morning in November 2013,[11] Emma, a master's degree student,
and Peter, a postdoctoral researcher, began their feeding routine in the Newborn
Pig Facility. This week Julie, one of the master's degree students in the group, had
provided each piglet with the name of a Nobel Prize winner and put name signs
with pictures of these famous scientists on the cages. Piglet A was named for
Albert Einstein, piglet R for Conrad *Röntgen*, piglet H for Andrew *Huxley*, and so
on. These names indicated both that the pigs were individuals and that they inescapably belonged to science: as substitutes for infants, they were disposable raw
material in the biographies of scientists and were jokingly treated as substitutes
for famous scientists, embodying their immortality.

In preparing the food for Huxley, Peter and Emma immediately observed that
he was limp and had a distended bowel. "Hey, sweetie," (*Hej, lille ven*) Emma
said calmly, as she gently put Huxley on the scale. Registering the weight of Huxley in the logbook, Peter noticed that the piglet had lost weight—which to him
was a sign of poor condition, as the experiment was based on the dominant
assumption in neonatology that growth indicates functional health. Thomas
entered the room and joined the discussion about Huxley. He decided to inject
rectal gel and water into the piglet's intestine to relieve its constipation. Peter
commented: "It's not well. I have to stick by what I usually say. The animals
should not suffer. This is *not* the intention. [If they do] then it isn't much fun."
Like every study in the Newborn Pig Facility, this one followed all ethical guidelines for professional conduct, but guidelines do not remove moral issues or
provide a clear answer on how, in this case, to improve Huxley's precarious situation. Thomas, Emma, and Peter agreed that the best thing for Huxley might be
to euthanize it right away to end its suffering, yet they also hesitated. More piglets than expected had had to be euthanized during this study, and if Huxley died
before the scheduled day of dissection, they would have to enroll a whole new
litter and run a new study to end up with a sufficiently large cohort. If Huxley
could not make it to the end of the study, a standardized death would produce
better samples than a nonstandardized one. In the latter case, Huxley's dying by
itself would result in organs that easily became too affected by death, and thus of
poor quality, when the dissection began. Consequently, keeping Huxley alive
was high gain (it might live to the end of the study) and high risk (it might die by
itself and result in poor samples). Displeased about the situation, Thomas commented, "We have put so many resources into a litter like this."

Their considerations were interrupted by Julie, who entered with an anaes-
thetized and sleeping piglet in her arms. This pig belonged to the litter that had

been enrolled in the Newborn Pig Facility four weeks earlier and had now reached its "kill day." Julie had taken on an enormous amount of work in caring for this litter and knew each of the piglets individually. Her toneless posture and unhappy face communicated her sadness about the impending killing of the pig in her arms. With a comforting smile, Peter said softly, "Should we call the grief counselor?" Although they all smiled at the joke, no one laughed at Julie. Based on their own experiences, everyone in the group was aware of the ambiguities of treating the piglets as both biological and biographical life. The care practices rescued the piglets from the "binary machine" (Bruns 2011, 75) of being either human or animal and placed them in an ambiguous zone of multiple identities. At the same time as the moral economy of the experimental practice defined the piglet in Julie's arms as "nongrievable" life (Butler 2016, 37), for the humans occupying the experimental space, the daily care practices momentarily turned it into grievable life.

When the researchers treated compromised piglets, they modeled a NICU situation in which almost everything will be done to secure an infant's survival and a considerable amount of suffering is tolerated because the infant has the potential of being healed and leaving the NICU with his or her parents. In that sense, the researchers "patientize the piglets" (Dam and Svendsen 2018, 360). The word "patient" comes from "pati," which means suffering, bearing, enduring, or permitting. When a pig substituted for the human patient, it shared suffering with infants in the NICU by enduring the pain of NICU infants. However, unlike the infants, the pig was never given the opportunity to leave the institutional setting. Rather, providing the pig with intensive care and attention became an integral part of the eventual death of the animal, not of treating it and letting it live. The hope was that the biological samples would embody the pig's care (as well as its pain), making the animal similar to the infants in the NICU.[12] But this way of constituting the piglets as convincing substitutive research subjects prompted questions among the researchers about the "ethics," as Marie phrased it, of balancing the good for the individual pig with the good for science.

As Huxley's respiration worsened, Thomas, Emma, and Peter decided that even if they chose not to euthanize the piglet, it would die very soon. Annoyed and sorry about the worsened situation, they decided to euthanize Huxley right away. By noon, Huxley and the pig in Julie's arms had been turned into more than eighty samples stored in the freezer.

GRANTING DEATH

One day in 2013, Thomas had been taking care of piglet M, which was not doing well. The pig had literally taken in the experimental setup, its gut inflamed due to its premature birth and the diet to which it had been randomly assigned. But Thomas had also taken in the precarious situation of the piglet. As he handed over his watch to Peter, Thomas stated in a serious tone, "I want you to treat M like it was your own son." Peter replied, "We do that already."[13] According to the protocol, piglet M was going to be killed in a matter of days, but that did not enter the discussion and thus did not strike any of the researchers as paradoxical. Similarly, Julie had cared intensively for piglets but had also engaged in turning them into samples. How was it possible for researchers to act as a (substituting) parent who treated pigs like kin and yet kill them a few days later?

In his discussion of sacrifice as a gift of death, Jacques Derrida (2008) explores the nature of the sacrifice by deconstructing the Judeo-Christian-Islamic myth of Abraham with Isaac at Mount Moriah. Drawing on the work of the Danish philosopher Søren Kierkegaard ([1843] 1983), Derrida proposes that by granting the gift of death, Abraham acted responsibly toward the absolute other (God) at the same time as he loved the one who was put to death (Isaac). It is this conflict between two contradictory responsibilities that constitutes the sacrifice (Derrida 2008, 64–66). Peter's and Thomas's care for piglet M and Julie's care for the anesthetized piglet in her arms epitomize this tension between their responsibility toward science and their love for the ones put to death. The contradiction between two responsibilities that, according to Derrida, constitutes sacrifice results in a tremendously fraught moment of treating the pig "like your own son" and then abstaining from treating the piglets as grievable humans who can escape suffering and killing. We may see this tension as a way to explore the boundaries of who and what falls within the norm of the human, and who and what does not. These boundaries are at the heart not only of human-animal relationships, but also of human-human relationships in which one part has been deemed "other" at various points in history (e.g., slaves in New World plantations, Jews in Nazi concentration camps, and civilians in Afghanistan in the U.S. war on terror). What the interactions in the Newborn Pig Facility help us see is that the framing that determines what falls within and what falls outside the norm of a human biographical, grievable life is constantly unsettled and transgressed by the very people who uphold it. "What are the ethics here?" Marie asks. The researchers' inability to reach closure points to an unresolved tension that is not simply experienced as an abstraction of two contrasting responsibilities—toward the piglets and toward science—as Derrida would have it. It is also a bodily tension between two kinds of substitution experiences: substituting for the pig by bearing responsibility for its personal well-being and substituting for the pig by bearing responsibility for turning it into health and welfare for humans.

Although the researchers articulate their moral engagement and resist closure, they do kill the piglets, thus embodying animal-use positions and enacting the human exclusionism so foundational to the Danish welfare state. In other words, in patientizing the piglets and caring for them as if they were their own children, the researchers turn each piglet into a "candidate for the human" (Bruns 2011, 45), thereby expanding the borders of humanity. In killing the piglets and turning them into samples, the researchers exclude the piglets from dying a human death and thus move them back into the category of nonhuman. These "shape-shifting" processes, as Sharp calls them (2019, 124–125), not only represent a shift in responsibility for the piglet as sentient kin and as research sample, but they also inform each other. Kinship does not run counter to sacrifice, as Radhika Govindrajan notes: "The death of an animal with whom people feel this embodied kinship creates a sense of loss and grief that is essential to making sacrifice *truly* a sacrifice. This is . . . the nature of sacrificial connection" (2018, 37). In the Newborn Pig Facility, the killing of cherished animals is a way of making kin in the present that connects the pig to future laboratory work and paves the way for improving nutrition for future preterm infants. The killing connects the pig to societal institutions and allows it to be appropriated by human collectives. Care as well as killing are constitutive of interspecies kinship (Dam et al. 2017), as expressed in Julie's sadness about the killing of her piglet. In these situations, the researchers expressed both their relatedness to the animals and their commitment to science.

As I noted in chapter 1, use fostered familiarity and intimacy with pigs. The use relations implied in caring for the piglets, killing them, and turning them into samples enact an interchange among pigs, researchers, and scientific institutions that is rooted in a long history of appropriating livestock for human needs. The ethnography from the Newborn Pig Facility reminds us of the affective aspects of this interchange and the moral worlds that are being created in human-animal intimacy. In appropriating the pigs by granting them death, the researchers walk the borders of the category of the human. Their moral negotiations are as much about their own belonging in a moral human community as they are about the humanness of the piglets in their care. In Sharp's words, "if laboratory life entails the (re)making of the animal for science, then, again, it involves the (re)making of the human, too" (2019, 151). By creating a moral context around the piglets as Peter, Thomas, and Emma did when deciding to euthanize Huxley, they strove to achieve the best good and sought to act virtuously by caring for Huxley as near human and killing it to complete its attachment to scientific institutions before it died on its own. In so doing they placed themselves in the "we" of concomitantly caring for the pig and using it as a possibility for the Danish welfare state collectivity by turning it into samples to generate education, scientific prestige, public-private partnerships, and future health for infants.

TURNING PIGLETS INTO SAMPLES

Lone, Morten, and Rikke worked intensely to equip a small room next to the room with the incubators for the last day of the study, which in the protocol was called euthanasia and sampling and was informally referred to as kill day or dissection day. This Friday in December 2009 was the fifth day in one of Lone's experimental weeks, and the ten piglets still alive from the latest litter were to be killed and turned into biological samples. For dissection days, the graduate student or postdoctoral researcher who had run the study gathered a team of four or five people to assist with the sampling. The person in charge brought candy, chips, or other goodies for the team, and very often the intensive work of dissecting the piglets took place in an atmosphere of both highly concentrated work and the excitement characteristic of putting an end to the experimental work—which would pave the way for the next phase of analyzing samples and beginning to write papers. There was also an "ordinary deadliness" (Wool 2015, 121) to the work of killing and dissecting. All of the researchers in the Newborn Pig Facility took part in dissecting almost every month—depending on the number of studies run—and thus killing, cutting, and sampling represented ordinary work rather than a heroic act of turning pigs into life for human infants.

In following different studies, I came to see the atmosphere on dissection day as partly related to the way the piglets had "behaved." When a number of piglets had been euthanized early (like Huxley), the expectations for the study results were moderate, and dissection was rather dull and ordinary work to be completed as quickly as possible. When a great number of piglets were in a very poor state yet still alive, and therefore could produce good data, the atmosphere was lively and full of both excitement about the study and relief about putting the piglets out of their misery and ending the researchers' intensive working days and nights. Both atmospheres point to dissection day as the turning point when the work of caring for the piglets was accomplished, moral issues about their suffering were resolved, and researchers hoped their long working hours' usefulness to both science and their own careers would be realized.

On this Friday, Lone and Morten sterilized the surfaces in the dissection room,[14] collected and put labels on cassettes and the small tubes in which tissue from the piglets was to be stored, prepared the scoring sheet on which they would note the condition and weight of the different organs of the animals, collected the knives they would need to use, filled a big container with ice, and prepared a nitrogen tank and put it on the table. Thomas and Jesper, a graduate student, arrived. Everyone put on white coats and clogs. These acts of preparation—together with Jesper's comment "Are we ready to put the show on the road?" and Lone's response, "Let's do it!"—marked the space and support the anthropological insights that a sacrifice cannot take place at just any time or in any place (Girard 1977; Hubert and Mauss 1968, 25). In the demarcated zone of the dissection room, the violence would take place at a specific time and on a selected number of prepared animals, thus facilitating the transformation of animals into scientific objects.

The killing repeatedly escaped my attention in the small dissection room. Instead, the administration of anesthesia stood out as the central and transformative act, which turned moving, sniffing, active piglets into docile, peaceful bodies that accepted the sacrificial killing. It was overwhelming to accompany

Rikke from the dissection room, equipped with ice and sterilized laboratory tools, down the corridor to the room with the piglets with its heat, noise, and smell of warm living bodies—many with diarrhea. Rikke prepared the anesthesia and opened the cage of the next piglet on her list. The piglet looked rather limp, and Rikke injected the anesthesia behind its ear. Nothing happened, and rather dissatisfied, Rikke mentioned that the anesthesia they were using at the moment worked slowly. Although the piglet was weak and unable to resist during the two minutes it took for the anesthesia to work, Rikke did not take it out of its cage until its body had collapsed and she was completely sure that it was asleep.

When we returned to the dissection room a minute later, everyone's attention was on the samples to be created. The piglet room and the dissection room spatially separated the two different appearances of the piglet, as sentient biographical life and nonsentient biological life. The ten-meter walk down the corridor from the piglet room with animals that smell and make sounds to the dissection room where silent, calm, and nonsentient piglet bodies reside convincingly configured the poison injected into the piglet's heart and the knives used for cutting the animal up as tools that remade the piglets into objects of science. Dissection day was not about unmaking the world, but about making it.

In the dissection room, there was usually lively and humorous conversation. Jesper moved the piglet from its box, put it onto a plate with ice, and took a blood sample from its heart. Lone grabbed the sample, commenting that it was "so strange that it is warm," and then corrected her blunder: "Oh, maybe it's not that strange." "No," Jesper replied laughingly, "it [the sample] is probably close to 37 degrees." This reminded Lone and the rest of us of the piglet's status as crossing the boundary between life and death: it was on its way to the freezer, but in this moment it was still a living and warm body. A second later, he injected poison, referred to as "the green squash," directly into the piglet's heart and then touched its chest to make sure that it was dead. Although Jesper was concentrating on his actions, no one else in the room paid much attention to the moment of death that definitively ended the corporeal exchange between the researchers and the piglets. All further activity in the room was dependent on and followed from this instant. As soon as death was a fact, Jesper cut the piglet's stomach open, filled it with ice, and took out the intestine, which was more than a meter long (see figures 2.3 and 2.4). He handed it to Morten, along with the piglet's other organs. Morten set the organs on an iced metal surface, placed a label with a number next to each organ, and photographed it. He then cut the intestine into many pieces and handed them to Rikke and Jesper. Five people worked intensely on transforming the full animal into labeled samples (see figure 2.5).

This detailed work on the piglet's body not only carved out the heart, liver, and intestine, but it also literally cut away the piglet as a sentient biographical life, abstracting it into medical categories and providing it with a new identity: it

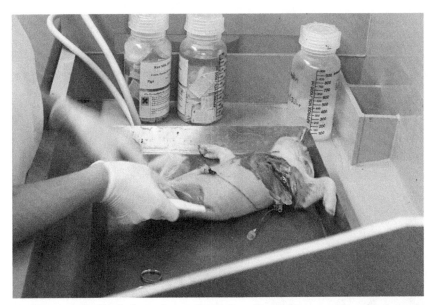

FIGURE 2.3. A dead piglet being dissected, Newborn Pig Facility, 2009. Photo by
the author.

shifted from a letter to a number, by which it would be known in all future scientific work to which it contributed. All the work the researchers put into feeding the piglets, attending to them, relieving their pain, and keeping them alive until this day was worth nothing if labels got mixed up or samples were not prepared properly or frozen immediately. As Peter commented during a dissection day in 2014, "You cannot be sloppy today. You need to be careful, otherwise all our efforts [with the living piglets] will be wasted."[15] In other words, to the researchers, the intimate care for the living piglets and the following euthanasia and sampling were mutually constitutive. Death paved the way for the next phase of research: the bench work that made up the first part of the long journey of moving the piglets into science; life for infants; and collaborative relations between the team, other research groups, and nutrition companies. The animal's entire body was cut up, sampled, and then remade into objects of science; it was disarticulated to rearticulate other bodies (Haraway 2008, 84).

This transformation of the living body into perpetually stored scientific objects represented a movement from pig bodies as "corporeal life" to tissue samples as "corporate life" (Parry 2004). In explaining their studies to an anthropologist colleague of mine, one of the senior researchers in the group referred to the freezers containing the pig samples as their "most precious" property. Death put the piglets on a track of future potential. The welfare state as receiver of this potential might not have been in Peter's thoughts on the intense morning of dissecting piglets. Nevertheless, the NEOMUNE research platform that included

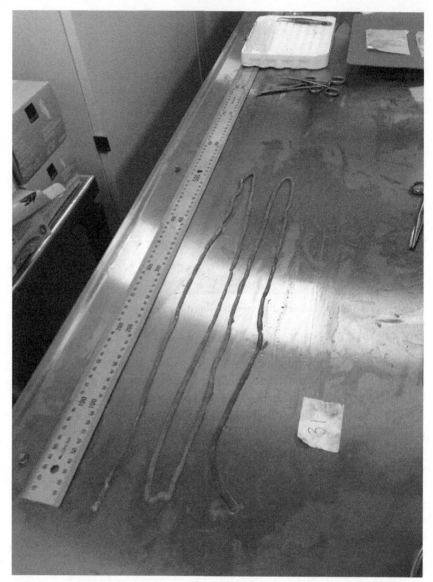

FIGURE 2.4. Intestine from a piglet, Newborn Pig Facility, 2013. Photo by Mie Seest Dam. (Credit: Mie Seest Dam.)

his postdoctoral position was funded by public money from the Danish Council for Strategic Research appropriated to "meet the challenges facing Danish society" and "ensure Denmark's position as a global frontrunner regarding welfare, wealth and science" (Danish Ministry of Higher Education and Science 2018). From this perspective, Peter's meticulous efforts to cut the brain out of the small

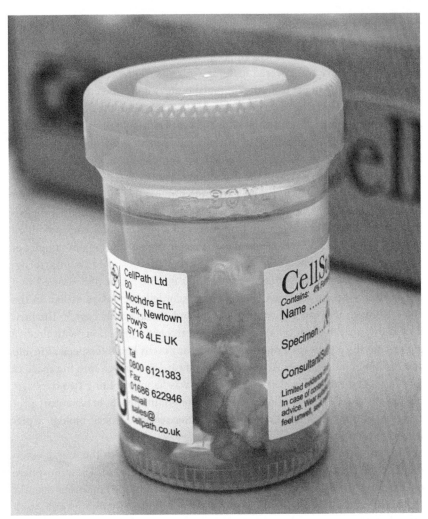

FIGURE 2.5. A sample of newly prepared brain tissue from a preterm piglet, Newborn Pig Facility, 2013. Photo by Mie Seest Dam. (Credit: Mie Seest Dam.)

piglet head consolidated the animal's kinship with the researchers and rendered visible the human-pig relationships at the heart of the Danish welfare state.

Not all dissection days included clear divisions between the piglets as first sentient and then nonsentient beings. In studies that lasted up to twenty-six days, dissection days tended to maintain the identity of the piglet as a sentient being. On one such day, I followed Julie, who had conducted many of the cognitive tests on the piglets and spent many hours with them during their twenty-six days in the lab. In the room of the live piglets she anesthetized one who had the Nobel Prize winner's name "Davisson," wrapped the sleeping creature in a cloth, and carried it like a small child in her arms. She said to me, "it is still my little pig that I have trained, but it has already become something completely different by now when it is anesthetized." On entering the dissection room, she carefully put the piglet on a tray and covered its body with a cloth. Marie told me that the cloth protected the piglet from the bright laboratory light, and covering its body "also just feels right." The practice of moving the piglet into the dissection room and preparing it for killing positioned it as a sentient biographical life ("my little pig," to be wrapped and protected) and literally hid its sentience by turning it into a faceless laboratory object ("something completely different," to be covered by a cloth) upon arrival in the dissection room.

At some stage during the intense work of sampling the animals, Julie entered the room again and stopped to chat with Peter, who was cutting up a piglet's brain. He had detached the brain from the skull and placed the empty skull on the table while he concentrated on the important work of cutting out samples of the brain. Looking at the skull, which was intact with eyes and hair, Julie recognized that this was Röntgen. She grabbed her mobile phone and showed us a one-minute video of Röntgen that she had recorded a few days earlier. In the video Röntgen was eagerly running around and sniffing in its cage.[16] The incident shows that it is not only during the researchers' interactions with the live piglets that the piglets for a moment come to appear as kin. Interspecies kinship and the biographical dimension of the pig's life are also woven into the space of carving out scientific samples (e.g., Röntgen was happily sniffing two days ago, but now its empty skull lies on the table). Throughout the whole laboratory process, substitution practices bind together the nonsentient generic biological piglet and the sentient biographical piglet.

The activities of killing, dissecting, and sampling spell out the moral lesson that the value of a pig's life is always lower than that of a human. The atmosphere on dissection day was often thick with both pig materiality and humorous remarks that testified to the "dilemmatic enterprise" of killing (Holmberg 2008, 330). One day during December 2009 as someone entered the dissection room, Morten shouted, "Welcome to the slaughterhouse!" Tina, an animal technician, commented: "You say 'slaughter.' Yesterday I said to my friend: 'Tomorrow we are going to murder pigs [dræbe grise],' and she answered: 'Can't you say that you put them down [aflive dem]?' 'No,' I said, 'we murder them [dræber grise].'" Rikke, who was labeling pieces of intestine, interrupted: "No, you are wrong. What we do is that we put them down." While the three of them disagreed about how to describe the act that had just happened, they also laughed. Lone grabbed a small container and jokingly begged Morten, "May I have my piece?" "You vulture!" Rikke commented ironically. Lone got her piece of intestine, put the container in her pocket, and left for the cell lab.[17]

If it is true that irony "names the recognition that one is subject to multiple and possibly competing, contradictory, or incommensurable aims, claims, intensions, desires, or commitments" (Lambek 2015, 20), the irony that loomed large in the laboratory points to the ethical scene that unfolds in the daily routines of care and killing. We might conceptualize this ethical scene as a "moral laboratory" (Mattingly 2014) in which the researchers strive to express and connect the multiple identities and valuations of piglet and human lives that become urgent in care and killing. In the laboratory, killing piglets abstracted the animals, turning them into units of liver, heart, and intestine. Yet in response to such abstractions, sentient and animate piglets lurked in the wings, together with their killers. The figure of the piglet as a pet to be "put down" in a clinical environment as an act of compassion (as Rikke would have it), a production animal to be "slaughtered" (as indicated in Morten's comment), and a being to be "murdered" (as Tina argued), made present the veterinary clinic, the pork producing industry, and the legal field of human rights. Each verb suggested a specific moral framing of the substitute. The joking conversation thereby sustained the view that the identity of the benign research clinician fighting disease goes hand in hand with that of the butcher who creates good food from "nongrievable" life, the murderer who kills grievable life, and the vulture that scavenges the meat of its victims. This vulture is ready to consume all sorts of pig: intestine, meat, and knowledge.

This humorous, yet fraught, moment illuminates what Sharp refers to as "the wrestling associated with moral conundrums" (2019, 8–9). Each identity, which gained presence in the joking interaction, has a different emotional valence. The clinician emphatically cares for human bodies that represent grievable lives, thus implicitly picturing piglets as patients. The butcher skillfully handles nongrievable carcasses, thus treating piglets as food for human consumption. While both of these identities stay within the boundaries of the law and in different ways make humans thrive, the murderer operates outside the law and kills human grievable lives, thus treating piglets as having the same moral standing as humans. All three researcher identities have an uncanny (*unheimlich*) side:[18] frightening and strange, yet simultaneously familiar.

Sharp writes that all researchers throughout their careers "ask themselves whether experimental practices cause undue harm; whether the quest for knowledge is worth the experimentation of other creatures; and under what circumstances, and with what species or specific animals, they should call a halt to their research" (2019, 149). The researchers' joking about the right words for the act of killing reflected the questions what makes us do this, and who are we when we do it? In his discussion of sacrifice, Derrida points to Abraham's silence when he decides to kill Isaac, and with Kierkegaard, Derrida argues that irony is a form of silence that provides a response without responding (2008, 74). We may see the joking as doing exactly that: it represented a collective reflection on who the researchers were when they brought about death in the laboratory, but it did not provide a clear answer or take sides. In the researchers' irony, I sense the intertwinement of sociomaterial and moral and affective practices that make pigs sacrificeable substitutes. This intertwinement revealed the pigs' multiple relationships with human beings and the many possible identities of both parties.

THE DISAPPEARANCE OF MONKEYS FROM DANISH RESEARCH LABS

The researchers kept reminding me that using pigs as model animals and killing them at the end of the study is closely connected to the routine slaughtering of about twenty-six million pigs every year in Denmark. In 2018, Denmark exported 1,911,850 tons of pork (Danish Agriculture and Food Council July 2019, 23). As Vinciane Despret notes, when animal bodies are measured in tons of meat for human consumption—rather than referred to as bodies or deceased beings—a translation has taken place that invisibilizes the meat's origin in animals and the violent act leading to animal death (2016, 81–87). Turning pigs into killable and nongrievable lives to become "roast pork," "chops," "shanks," or "schnitzels" involves a "'deanimalization' of the animal" (quoted, 83). In the Newborn Pig Facility, the fact that industrial farming rendered pigs killable provided an unshakable ethical foundation for the researchers' work. It is precisely the pigs' biological proximity to humans and the social acceptance of their deaths that make them near human. In contrast to the human, the near human can be killed. To illustrate the politics involved in making killable and its historical contingency, I turn to a story about the last research monkeys on Danish territory, a case study that Lene Koch and I have researched.[19] The disappearance of monkeys from Danish and other European laboratories around 2000 did not put an end to primate research but moved it abroad. Thus, the public outcry over what was deemed to be morally problematic research on nonhuman primates was hypocritical as the research continued, although not on Danish ground. Nevertheless, the departure of monkeys from laboratories around 2000 indicates a profound change in the European moral landscape of animal experimentation and provides insights into the trend that favored using the porcine model.

In the 1920s and 1930s, nonhuman primates played a prominent role in the development of biomedical sciences and therapeutics (Clarke 1998; Druglitrø 2016; Friese and Clarke 2012; Haraway 1989). Their close genetic and evolutionary proximity to humans made them key in vaccine production, toxicology, xenotransplantation, and reproductive science. In the 1950s, nonhuman primates were used extensively in biomedical research laboratories in Denmark. In the 1980s, a leading lab in the field of Danish biological psychiatric research acquired a group of capuchin monkeys to be used in research aimed at reducing the serious side effects of medication for schizophrenia. Research from the laboratory had already become groundbreaking internationally and played a significant role in the success of Lundbeck, a Danish pharmaceutical company. The monkeys were transported to Denmark via facilities in the United Kingdom and the United States. In Denmark, the monkeys were housed at a psychiatric hospital. They were placed in a basement lab in individual, small cages[20] and used for experiments several times a week. One group of experiments required the administration of amphetamine to induce psychotic-like behavior in the monkeys, thus turning them into a model for psychosis. After this, they were given increasing doses of antipsychotic drugs to see when this would counter the psychosis. Various drugs—most of them dopamine agonists or antagonists—were studied during the experiments. In some cases, the monkeys were used for studies sponsored by the pharmaceutical industry, and in other cases the psychiatric hospital housing the laboratory financed the experiments. Some of the drugs tested had been produced by Lundbeck or Novo Nordisk, another Danish pharmaceutical company. The monkeys' placement in individual cages, where they could not touch each other, reflected the dominant view at the time that the animals were simply generic "nongrievable" biological lives, instrumentally valuable for serving human interests.

In the beginning of the twenty-first century, more than twenty years after the first group of capuchins arrived in the lab, the understanding of the close biological and social proximity between human and monkey made it increasingly morally unpleasant to use nonhuman primates in research in Europe. The Council of Europe and the EU had continued to emphasize the moral value of animals, and the EU was preparing new directives that stressed the ethical and practical problems of meeting the behavioral, environmental, and social needs of nonhuman primates in scientific procedures. This new piece of legislation would narrow the biomedical arenas in which the use of nonhuman primates would be permitted.[21] With these tightening regulations, nonhuman primates increasingly came to belong to the category of beings whose members the Nuremberg Code intended to protect from experimentation—those with almost as high a moral status as human beings. In Denmark, academic and industry researchers soon abandoned domestic research on nonhuman primates and began contracting with nonhuman primate centers and contract labs abroad.

As the monkey model was losing its value, the psychiatric laboratory found that the anticipated regulatory changes would make continued experiments with nonhuman primates on Danish soil too expensive. Also, the laboratory felt a need to present itself to the Danish public as an ethically responsible institution. The usual outcome of a decision to end lab experiments with animals is the killing of the animals. But that did not happen in this case. Following months of negotiations, the lab entered an alliance with the Danish Animal Welfare Society and Novo Nordisk with the aim of transferring the monkeys to a Danish zoo. The Danish Animal Welfare Society hired two specialists on nonhuman primates to write a report on the health and rehabilitation potential of the animals. The report concluded that the majority of the monkeys could be used for breeding purposes in a zoo. This possible future linked the monkeys to several long-term projects. One was an international attempt to produce capuchins in zoos that were bred to save the threatened species. Another was to use the new housing arrangement in the zoo as a living experiment for group-based housing for future nonhuman primates in overseas contract labs. The zoo, therefore, should not be mistaken for the wilderness, nor should rehabilitation be mistaken for freedom. No Danish zoo had capuchins at the time, and since some of the monkeys had been born in the wild, they were considered a valuable genetic resource. The report concluded that only the twelve males had the potential to regain their original natural characteristics, whereas the females were considered beyond repair and the damage to their mental and physical health irreversible. As a result, euthanasia of the females was deemed the ethically correct solution. One final killing act was needed to pave the way for more morally acceptable forms of control.

In the Danish press, the rehabilitation of research monkeys from the psychiatric hospital lab was presented as part of a public rescue mission. In 2012, when Lene and I visited the zoo to which the capuchins had been transferred in 2004, the zoo director told us that the cage designed for the monkeys was made to resemble a tree-top, in keeping with capuchins' natural habitat. As zoo animals, the ideal was for monkeys to live as long as possible and die from old age, and thus they gained an open future. Their transfer to the zoo was presented as a moral project, a way to do them good. In one of the many newspaper articles about the monkeys, a representative from Novo Nordisk explained that killing lab animals after experiments was "old fashioned" and that animals should never be considered "pure instruments. . . . Monkeys are living individuals whom we have used to serve man for more than 20 years. The least we can do is to make sure that the last phase of their lives is as good as possible."[22] Such views were further elaborated on in our interviews with other Novo Nordisk representatives. One pointed to the similarity between humans and monkeys: "When we use animals, we must treat them with respect. They are living beings, and as human beings we are closely linked to the animals." The current head of bioethics at Novo Nordisk pointed to guilt and responsibility as main arguments for financing the rehab project: "Those monkeys have been through a lot of cruelty, they have had awful lives, and we have a duty to help now." Another Novo Nordisk manager agreed, saying that "Novo tested a range of substances on these animals and felt obliged to help." In these interviews, the monkeys gained a biography. They were provided with a past and subjective experiences that had been imprinted on their bodies and became arguments for their new moral value and need for rehabilitation. By providing the monkeys with sentience and biography, they became lives that could be lost and grieved.

The remarkable transfer of the last research monkeys on Danish territory spells out the potentiality path of the pig substitute in the moral landscape of animal experimentation. In this landscape, it is not only the pig's similarity to human biology but also the public consensus when it comes to its sacrificial nature that continues to pave its way into Danish research laboratories. Despite the many ways in which pigs are turned into near human in laboratory practices, they do not lose their identity as just a pig, positioned between food and pharmaceutical production (Sharp 2014, 81). By eating pork, Danes are already implicated in its destiny as a killable animal. As Professor Per remarked to me, the cutting up of millions of pigs for food makes it publicly acceptable to cut up pigs for science. Conversations in the Newborn Pig Facility leaned on the dominant cultural logic of seeing the pig as expendable and treating its death as an "ethical non-issue" (Wolfe 2010, 49). The phrase "just a pig" (see prologue) provides the animal with a moral flexibility that the monkeys lost when they moved away from near humanness toward a morally valuable monkeyness. It may be that most people think of monkeys as de facto near human, but my juxtaposition tells us differently. The Danish research monkeys were near human, but they lost that status when they were reanimalized and regained monkeyness. In the zoo, this monkeyness continued to coexist with instrumentalization, although the animals undoubtedly were exposed to less brutality than they had been in the lab. In their new collective cages, the monkeys moved closer to the moral value of the human, as they acquired a biographical life and an open future. Concurrently, the transfer from narrow, individual cages in the lab to the spacious cage in the zoo with access to an outdoor island also implied a closeness to their animal nature.

The comparison between the end of using research monkeys on Danish ground and the continued use of pigs in medical research in Denmark highlights how the flexibility of the pig makes it possible for human caregivers to turn it into intimate kin and make it suffer and treat it as an expendable animal on the day of dissection, although the latter actions are saturated with moral perils. In contrast to the monkeys, who lost their potential as substitutive research subjects, the pigs' identity as sacrificial substitutes for humans paves the way for them to move across species boundaries and become near human in laboratory practices.

THE TEMPORAL HORIZONS OF SACRIFICE

When Marie, in the opening quote in this chapter, notes that she always begins with the infants when she describes her work to strangers, she is ordering the relationships between infants and piglets in terms of original and substitute. If I based my account on such legitimating statements, substitution could be understood simply as a way of symbolically standing in for another being—as is also the case in some anthropological reflections on sacrifice (Smith and Doniger 1989). What the daily practices in the lab revealed, though, is that the substitute is itself in need of substitution. When researchers substitute for piglets, they engage in "relational extension" (Latimer 2013, 98) by acting as a proxy and taking a stance on the value of the piglets' lives. This involves thinking not only about what is good for the individual piglet, but also what is good for science— which one animal technician referred to as "the big picture" of completing studies, running an educational institution, fulfilling obligations in research collaborations, and contributing to infant health. Moreover, this tension between what is good for the pig and what is good for science involves a navigation between what one may accept within the experimental space and how strangers may look at it. Marie's caution about how she talks about her research illuminates the fact that woven into the ethical dilemmas I have unfolded in this chapter is the question of how invisible publics may judge the researchers' actions.

In the Newborn Pig Facility, drawing piglets into suffering and thus temporarily unmaking the world and causing moral perils for oneself is conceptualized as part of making the world. Consequently, as much as daily practices in the laboratory are about unsettling species boundaries by stepping into the position of the pig, they also involve actively drawing boundaries between the lesser worth of the pig and the higher worth of the human. In the interview in which Thomas reminded Mie and me of the researcher's "feel" for the animal ("How would you feel if your condition was like that [of the pig]?"), he also reflected upon the moral worth of both piglet and human researcher: "Is it true that the human is a unique species that has more worth than animals? I don't think so. I don't think that I have a right to exploit the animal, but I acquire the right because I can." He then made clear to us that "taking the right" was about creating health for preterm infants, thereby situating his actions within the unshakable moral economy of animal experimentation that unambiguously conditions the animal as a tool for human health. His reflections illuminate how the researchers are constantly trying to determine the acceptable way of handling piglet suffering in the context of both the animal's existential affinity with the human ("How would you feel?") and its identity as a tool for human health and potential ("taking the right"). As Julie's sadness about the impending killing of the pig in her arms also indicates, the researchers "know grief firsthand" (Despret 2016, 87), and resist moral closure. They accept that "exploitation," as Thomas called it, flows in the direction of the piglets, yet they never stop engaging with the moral ambiguities related to caring for and killing suffering animals. In Thomas's reflection, we sense neither a victorious statement about using piglets as research tools nor any regrets about his work life. After the interview, Thomas went back to his work with the piglets and a few days later helped with killing and dissecting them. His reflections capture my initial confusion about the pervasive animal-use positions in the lab and the researchers' treatment of the piglets as fellow beings. As Sara Ahmed states, "affection and instrumentality can be different threads woven together in the same story about use" (2019, 7). In walking the borders between animal death and human life in the tactile laboratory space that constitutes the frontier of translational medicine, the researchers affectionately strive to do well for the piglets, while at the same time instrumentalizing them to produce infant health. Their simultaneous acts of care and use unfold alongside questions about the ethics of animal suffering and uniqueness of human worth.

The researchers' virtuous acts of caring for vulnerable piglets and "the big picture" of improving health for vulnerable infants eventually made me recognize not only moral peril, but also the temporal orientations inherent in the sacrificial exchange and the interspecies kinship it materializes. Although individual piglets die on kill day, the researchers' continuous work on their bodies provides them with an afterlife and establishes a temporal path that is indeterminate: no one knows whether five, ten, or twenty years will pass before the piglet studies might have an effect on infant health. Here, temperature played a significant role in destabilizing the dichotomy between life and death and creating a sense of suspense (Hoeyer 2017, 206–207) as frozen samples could be revisited, exchanged, analyzed with new technologies or in other ways potentialized in the future. This indeterminate temporal horizon comes close to what the literary theorist Frank Kermode refers to as "aevum" (2000, 70), which in medieval Latin describes a mode of existence between worldly time and eternity. In Christian philosophy, the aevum was occupied by angels (71–82, 194). Whereas the loss of a child in the NICU was mourned as the loss of a potential future, the controlled death of piglets in the Newborn Pig Facility and the freezing of specimens initiated their future and included them anew in the welfare state collectivity. Having entered the temporality of angels (the aevum), the piglets were dead and no longer of worldly time, yet through the bench work of the researchers they had the potential for acting in worldly time, creating value for future infants, and becoming immortal, as suggested by being named after Nobel Prize winners.

Although the piglets had short lives measured in calendar days, the temporality that surrounded their death provided them with a more spacious future and a longer prospect than many humans have. Death completed the interspecies kinship tie between the piglets and the infants, which the research was all about, and made the piglets communal through their connection to "the big picture" of "running the machine." As dead samples, the piglets carried the hope of becoming deathless angels, tying science and health together for the welfare state collectivity. In the end, substitution not only played out in human-animal relationships in the experimental practices; it also came in the form of angel animals that, beyond death, continue to act in time and assist humans. The instrumentalization of pig lives in daily experimental practices testifies to prevailing anthropocentric bioethics that praise the newborn child as an "icon of life" (Morgan 2009). With its plastic potential for emerging humanness, the piglet substitute has the future of the human infant built into it. The sacredness of humanness seems to absorb everything that flows down the great chain of being, in particular the piglet that is unmade and remade to become health for human infants.

At the same time as the human infant in the NICU represents an icon of life, that infant does not possess the consciousness and cognitive abilities claimed to differentiate the human from the pig according to anthropocentric bioethics. Intellectually and cognitively, the premature infant is similar to, rather than different from, the premature piglet. So how is the life of precarious human infants negotiated in the NICU? What notions of human sociality, potential, and fulfillment come to the fore when infants enter life far too early? These are the questions to which I return in chapter 3.

3 · TREATING
Infants at the Margins of Life

From my position two meters from the incubator, it takes a while before I can distinguish Emily's tiny body of 450 grams behind the wires. This morning she has been taken out of the incubator, and two nurses are tinkering with her respirator, which causes her oxygen saturation numbers on a screen next to the incubator to drop and the device to emit loud beeps. On a hospital bed next to the incubator, Emily's mother is pumping milk, and Emily's father sits next to his wife. I stay behind the neonatologist who is to inspect Emily, and I realize that my reluctance to approach her incubator is not only about avoiding standing in the way of the doctor. In addition, my fear of transgressing on the privacy of Emily and her parents holds me back.

In the Newborn Pig Facility, I would also be careful not to stand in the way of the researchers, but there I had no problem walking close to the incubator-like cages, observing the piglets, commenting on them, and taking photos of them. In that setting, the sow was absent. The piglets belonged to the research team, and once the team had let me in, this implied that I had full rights to access the animals. I never thought of the privacy and subjectivity of the piglets as something I should respect in my way of approaching them. It may seem jarring and inappropriate to bring my experience in the Newborn Pig Facility into a discussion of the neonatal intensive care unit (NICU). Of course, one cannot object that there is a difference between the human clinic and the animal lab. Nevertheless, in this chapter I suggest that juxtaposing the two sites exposes what it takes to become a certain form of life. In particular, my methodology of juxtaposition (explained in more detail in the introduction) has helped me see the role of kinship in constituting the child as grievable and losable. Through my first days of fieldwork in the NICU, I notice that when the parents are not in the room when I enter in the company of doctors and nurses, my experience of the infant and its sphere of privacy is more similar to my experience in the pig facility. With the parents absent, the infant tends to appear as a belonging of the hospital to which he or she is connected through tubes and monitors, and it is easier for me to look at the child and question the doctors about his or her condition. When the parents are in the room or when a teddy bear or a picture of siblings decorate the incubator, the child's embeddedness in relations beyond the hospital materialize. This morning, Emily's parents' presence on the bed certainly makes me think about how their lives have changed from one moment to the next, when a normal pregnancy turned into a preterm birth in week twenty-five. I identify with them and sense their sorrow and distress. Will they be able to bring their daughter home? Their presence in the room turns Emily into a subject belonging to them. As I hesitantly walk closer to Emily, I feel that I have set foot in their territory.

The role of the parents in contributing to the infant's status as a person is also present in other and very profound ways. As I look at the neonatologist's grave expression as she inspects Emily, I am reminded of a conversation during the doctors' round an hour earlier on this Monday morning. Tina, a senior doctor from the weekend team, reported that Emily, who suffers from necrotizing enterocolitis (NEC), had to have an immediate operation as her NEC reached a critical stage and caused bowel perforation. Dr. Tina told her colleagues that she had had a productive conversation with Emily's parents about their choices: either carrying out the operation or withdrawing treatment, which would have meant that Emily would die. In response to this information, the head of the clinic, Dr. Mads, asked if the "background and situation" of the parents would point in the direction of not carrying out the operation. With his use of the phrase "background and situation," he was hinting at the social and emotional resources of the family. As we saw in the case of Cheung (see the introduction), clinicians do not consider it right to save an infant if the child is not wanted by the parents. In the doctors' round, Dr. Tina said that the parents' situation did not point toward withdrawing treatment, but the conversation helped the parents realize how critically ill Emily was and discuss the possibility of not continuing.

Dr. Tina's conversation with the parents illustrates the distribution of responsibility in life-and-death decision making.[1] In Denmark, doctors have the authority to decide to abstain from lifesaving treatment in cases where patients are irreversibly dying, severely disabled or in a persistent vegetative state, or not irreversibly dying but in a state where the physical consequences of disease or treatment are considered very severe or painful (*meget alvorlige og lidelsesfulde*) (Danish Health Authority 2012).[2] Yet doctors are seriously committed to involving patients and relatives in decision making. The guideline in effect in the region where this NICU's hospital is located says that in the case of infants born before twenty-six weeks gestation, the doctors in collaboration with the parents must continuously estimate "indications for treatment" and that "a prenatal conversation with the parents is crucial." The guideline further stresses that "the assessment is made by a doctor and possibly a nurse and must take into account the parents' wishes, their opportunities, and the individual child's maturity, and possible diseases" (Capital Region, n.d.). According to these guidelines, doctors are simultaneously committed to exercising medical authority in the assessment of infants' viability and to considering parental preferences and "opportunities," thus attending to the overall situation and happiness of families.[3]

The guidelines reflect the fact that Denmark does not have a strong right-to-life movement.[4] The state-financed health services in Denmark offer legal and subsidized abortions until the end of the twelfth week of pregnancy. Between the thirteenth and twenty-second weeks, abortion needs to be sanctioned by the regional Joint Council of Abortion. The termination of a pregnancy at this stage is paid for by the Danish state if the potential child is expected to have a serious health problem and/or the prospective parents are expected to have a low quality of life as a result of the child's condition. This approach spills over into life-and-death decision making in the NICU. There, choices about whether and how an infant born before twenty-six weeks gestation should receive treatment are made not purely on the basis of saving life at all costs but take into account the presumed quality of life of the infant and his or her family, if complications of continued treatment lead to a life of very severe disability. Assessments of the infant's brain function and future ability to think, feel, move, and relate to others are significant, especially in these discussions.

As the neonatologist guides me closer to Emily's incubator and I see Emily's miniature body and the ostomy bags containing a tiny bit of green liquid, I realize the enormous work of substituting for her. Although the situation appears so much more devastating than caring for piglets in the laboratory, in both sites the professionals' substitution engages the sociomaterial replacement of biological processes in the body (in Emily's case, using respirators, medications, and ostomy bags) and the moral and affective practice of "being alongside" (Latimer 2013) neonates by performing partial connectedness to their world and relations. Before Dr. Tina had a conversation with Emily's parents over the weekend, she had read through Emily's medical record, interpreted the newly arrived laboratory results, looked at the scans, and used her long experience in neonatology to optimize the NICU environment's replacement of Emily's bodily functions. And when Dr. Tina talked to Emily's parents, she imagined their future and sought to answer difficult questions about Emily's viability and prospects. In Dr. Tina's care, the sociomaterial replacement and the moral and affective practice of connecting to Emily and her parents' situation are interwoven.

Questions of viability in the context of the beginning of human life enter the terrain of selective reproduction. Such reproduction constitutes political acts of letting some lives into or out of society and necessarily implies negotiations about what it takes to be a member of society. It covers a range of practices around the world and throughout history, from abandonment of children to eugenic selection in Europe and the United States in the early twentieth century and later techniques such as ultrasound scans, the abortion of fetuses, and genetic testing to intervene in unborn life.[5] In Emily's NICU room, profound questions about what constitutes a good life—and a good death—are unfolding before our eyes. These questions involve paying attention to the life of the family and the belonging of the infant to the family and welfare state. In what follows, I refer to these negotiations as the "work of viability" (Christoffersen-Deb 2012, 587). What qualifies and what does not qualify as an infant on the verge of a life to be saved and become a member of society? And how are these negotiations made manifest through daily acts of substitution?

BIOLOGICAL AND BIOGRAPHICAL LIFE IN THE NICU

In the context of life sciences, intriguing anthropological studies have rendered visible the ambiguous meanings of bodily material when human specimens are collected (Morgan 2009, Olejaz 2017) and bits and parts of bodies travel beyond their source and continue to show a potential for human personhood (Hoeyer 2013). In the context of technologies aimed at caring and monitoring bodies in early and late life, other ethnographies demonstrate the biopolitical forces and the lived experiences that shape the becoming or erosion of human personhood in the realm of the liminal (Gammeltoft 2014; Kaufman 2005; Lock 2002; Taylor 2008). Despite these studies' sensitivity toward personhood as fabricated, they focus solely on human personhood and thus they tend to treat the human being as their self-evident starting point for an investigation of personhood. In this chapter, I take inspiration from multispecies investigations that extend ethnography beyond the human realm. Yet where multispecies ethnography has uncovered the ecological interconnectedness of humans and other species, I uncover the social, temporal, and spatial configurations of neonate life in the NICU and the Newborn Pig Facility. By following my initial juxtaposing move, when I hesitantly approached Emily's incubator and realized the absence of this hesitation in my interactions with research pigs, I show that care for piglets may bring to the fore the "person" and biographical life of the animal, just as care and decision making in the NICU may bring to the fore the biological organism of the infant.

In engaging these juxtapositions between lab and clinic, I am particularly interested in the associations gained and shed when human and pig neonates move between biological and biographical life, when they come to contain amounts of both, and when the biological and the biographical interact or are brought into tension. My movements between the NICU and the Newborn Pig Facility expose the fact that substitution practices produce a qualified biographical life by placing the infant in social relationships (to kin and the welfare state), imbuing the infant with an open future, and expecting the infant to gain the mental and physical capacities of moving in an open space. Based on these observations, I argue that the symbiopolitics at stake in connecting the lives of piglets to the lives of infants is not only a question of moving across knowledge and cow colostrum from animal lab to clinic, as discussed in chapter 1. It also involves a moral division between human and pig that is present in the social, temporal, and spatial constitution of their lives and deaths. Turning piglets into research tools and making them bioavailable is thus enabled by detaching the piglets from the mother sow, housing them in a state institution for a limited period of time, as well as by placing infants in kinship and linking them to both open-ended futures and a home outside state institutions. In other words, saving the lives of human infants with the aim of turning them into take-home babies cannot be dissociated from housing research animals in laboratories. Even constituting mere biological life is a social, temporal, and spatial achievement.

Most infants in the NICU are successfully treated and leave the hospital with their parents. In this light, it may seem a bit misleading that I take my empirical point of departure in situations where there is a crisis of viability. Nevertheless, in the following discussion I highlight these extraordinary cases because they more clearly show us how the different aspects of biological and biographical life are being negotiated, put in tension, or conjoined, as well as how uncertainty about the future exposes questions about initiating, continuing, or withdrawing treatment. Below in the chapter, I place life-and-death decision making in the NICU in the context of Danish human reproductive politics from the 1930s to the present. In the beginning of the twentieth century, eugenic policies were part of the social reforms that built up the welfare state, and in the latter half of that century, state-financed prenatal diagnostics became an indispensable part of public health and gained overwhelming public support. This historical perspective demonstrates that for nearly a century, the exclusion of specific unborn lives has been part and parcel of welfare state policies that aim to provide equal life opportunities for citizens and build and maintain a sustainable society. My claim is that in Danish reproductive politics—with regard to both humans and pigs—the exclusion of certain lives is seen as a necessary condition for the creation of an equal society.

KINSHIP AND THE FABRICATION OF A BIOGRAPHICAL LIFE

Hannah and her twin sister, Elisabeth, were born at full term. Elisabeth was completely healthy, but Hannah suffered from a severe heart complication that was diagnosed at birth. Each parent had a child from an earlier marriage, and the mother had been through in vitro fertilization (IVF) to conceive the twins. In the company of the nurse, I entered Hannah's room and immediately noticed her sallow skin and the blue spots on the stomach due to her poor circulation. Above her cradle was a poster with her birth date and the names of her mother, father, and siblings, which staff members always make for every new child entering the NICU. During a child's stay, drawings from siblings or cousins, photos of

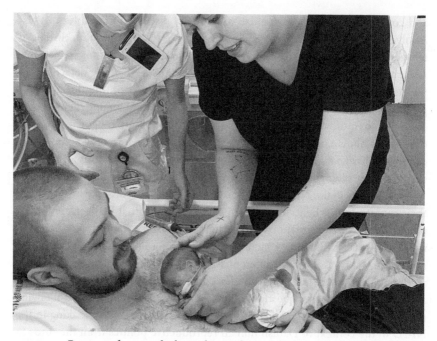

FIGURE 3.1. Parents and a nurse facilitate skin-to-skin contact between a prematurely born infant and her father, Copenhagen NICU, 2021. Photo by Linda Svenstrup Munk. (Credit: Copenhagen University Hospital.)

the parents, and gifts such as teddy bears may decorate the incubator, crib, or space next to the machinery that surrounds the child. Just as the presence of Emily's parents connected her to a family history and a world beyond the hospital, these decorations contribute to providing the infant with a biographical life by placing the newly arrived infant in kin relationships—which also implied that the infant's kin gain new identities of mother, father, sibling, or grandparent. The longer the stay in the NICU, the more objects and decorations will appear and strengthen the tie of the infant to people and places outside the NICU. Hannah had arrived only the day before, and her cradle was still undecorated with drawings made by her family members.

This emphasis on the child's kinship and connections to home also came to the fore in other ways. In the NICU, body-to-body contact was seen as crucial to establishing connections between infants and parents. Usually the nurse would put an infant on the chest of his or her mother or father for a short while before returning the infant to the incubator. This was referred to as "getting out" (*at komme ud*) and was usually an event that the parents were excited about and looked forward to (see figure 3.1). "Getting out" also signified that the infant was on his or her way to graduate to rooms with less intensive care and more "open" beds, and a life in which the infant could freely be moved around and come closer to his or her parents (Layne 1996). In this way, "getting out" enacted what treatment in the NICU was aimed at—namely, making it possible for the infant to start a life outside the hospital and enter the place where parents, siblings, and friends had their everyday lives.

Next to the poster with Hannah's name and the names of her family members was a postcard, also made by staff members, with an imprint of Hannah's foot. It said, "To big brother from Hannah." The presence of the card indicated that her older brother had not yet visited her. The parents' bed next to the cradle was empty, but a few minutes later, Hannah's father entered with Hannah's healthy twin, Elisabeth.

During the following days, the father was present in the ward and engaged in many conversations with the heart physician who monitored Hannah's condition and planned an upcoming operation. His wife was in the maternity ward and did not show up. The doctors and nurses found this very problematic. In one conversation, the nurse approached the father and said: "I'm concerned about the attachment between mother and child. I think the mother should be present as much as possible." The father explained that his wife was devastated by Hannah's illness and was crying constantly. Later in their conversation, the nurse said: "Hannah has heard her mother's voice all through the pregnancy, and it is important that she continues hearing that voice. . . . If the mother hasn't bonded with the child during the stay in hospital, it can get difficult when Hannah returns home—and even more difficult if Hannah does not come home." The "it" that "can get difficult" seemed to refer not only to the relationship between Hannah and her mother but to the entire situation and emotional well-being of the family. In response, Hannah's father said: "If it becomes a long and complicated trajectory—and it will—then I have decided that it [continued treatment] should not be at all costs. At some point, a decision needs to be made about either one way or the other way [at det enten skal gå den ene vej eller den anden vej]. Because in the end, you get so fed up with the hospital [the father mimes a strangulation], and life needs to go on."

This conversation communicated the "attachment imperative" (Navne, Svendsen, and Gammeltoft, 2018) in the clinic as a politics of belonging that treats attachment between children and parents as the ground on which to carry out and make meaningful the daily care practices and the difficult life-and-death decisions for infants on the fringes of life. Although staff members were dissatisfied with the absence of Hannah's mother, the conversation also showed strong alignment between the father and the staff. The word "death" was not spoken by the nurse or Hannah's father, but through euphemisms they both addressed the possibility of Hannah's dying and the importance of securing a good family life. In particular, Hannah's father referred to the social and emotional "costs" of staying in the hospital with a very sick child and caring for a very sick child through his or her life. In this dialogue, the nurse and Hannah's father not only substituted for

Hannah by stepping into her position to ask what kind of life she may lead. They also stepped into the position of the family. Hannah's father was concerned about the two older siblings (the brother had been in despair at Hannah's situation and did not want to see her), and he was comforted by the fact that Elisabeth was healthy and would come home with him and his wife. He said that Hannah might have perished during his wife's pregnancy, but "now she has made it so far and should have a chance." Staff members did not condemn the father for alluding to the possibility of withdrawing treatment if Hannah's situation worsened. Rather, they saw the fact that he raised this possibility as a positive indication that he understood Hannah's precarious situation. Moreover, his presence in the clinic and his support of Hannah's being given a chance was to them an act that confirmed Hannah as a qualified biographical life rooted in loving relations.

The NICU's emphasis on a good family life and the infant's kin relationships resonates with Danish reproductive politics. While state-financed access to specific forms of infertility treatment was introduced in the late 1980s, in 2006 the Danish Fertility Law was revised to require that IVF clinics assess what was referred to as candidates' "ability to parent" (Section § 6a). This requirement of parenting ability was extended in 2010, after an incident in which a child born through state-financed fertility treatment had to be admitted to public care because the parents were assessed as being unable to provide acceptable rearing and life conditions for the child.[6] Parenting ability also appears in other guidelines regarding reproduction. For instance, the Danish Health Authority (2009, 65–70) recommends that women with severe social and psychological problems should be offered counseling before conception and that women with alcohol and drug problems should be informed about the availability of abortion.[7] These policies express a specific biopolitics in which high-quality universal care coexists with a readiness to withdraw treatment or terminate pregnancy based on ideas about a meaningful life for the infant and the family.

Dr. Tina's conversation with Emily's parents and the dialogue between the nurse and Hannah's father echo Judith Butler's notion of precariousness as the "condition of being conditioned" (2016, 23). These families' situations acknowledge that neonates are dependent on "a social network of hands" (14) in the form of a well-functioning family and societal support. In contrast to the situation of Cheung's parents (see the introduction), both Hannah's and Emily's parents were obviously Danish citizens (white, Scandinavian-looking people who spoke Danish and had Danish names), and thus societal support in the form of public health care that would subsidize costly operations and lifelong support was taken for granted among both clinicians and parents. What was not taken for granted was the family situation. In the conversation between Hannah's father and the nurse, the fear that long hospitalizations of a severely disabled child might constitute too much of a burden for the family raised questions about the worthiness of Hannah's life, based on an acknowledgment of interdependence as a condition of life. Taking this interdependence seriously, Hannah's father and the nurse allowed space for the possibility that Hannah might turn into a losable life.

In Butler's exploration of grievable life, she does not distinguish between nongrievable life and losable life. In her work, nongrievability constitutes losability. In the NICU, however, withdrawing treatment from very precarious infants did not make them nongrievable. Such children were losable, but they were still worth grieving. When infants hover between life and death and continued treatment may result in severe disabilities, the parents' situation and wishes contribute to constituting the infant as either nonlosable and grievable or losable and grievable, paving the way for either its inclusion in life or its exclusion from it.

SOCIAL RELATIONS: PLACING THE CHILD IN THE FAMILY AND THE WELFARE STATE

If parental attachment and functional family life are considered essential to constituting precarious infants as viable and nonlosable people, what happens when infants on the very margins of life have vulnerable kin relations?

At the daily medical round a few days before Hannah was admitted to the NICU, the group was informed that an alcoholic pregnant woman, who also smoked cannabis on a regular basis, had been admitted to the hospital and was expected to give birth soon.[8] The father was an alcoholic, too. The woman had asked for an abortion when she was seventeen weeks pregnant, yet she had not managed to make a formal application to the Joint Council of Abortion although she strongly wanted to abort. The woman was estimated to be in her twenty-fifth week of gestation. The group was also informed that the woman had a fourteen-year-old daughter who had been taken into state care immediately after birth. The senior resident initiated the discussion of the case by saying, "This infant is to be treated like all other infants, apart from the fact that it shall not be given active treatment." In further explaining his stance, he stated that abstaining from active treatment corresponded with the ability-to-parent guideline. He thereby explicitly imported the logic of a guideline for IVF treatment into life-and-death decisions in the NICU and implicitly (and maybe unwittingly) drew on the guideline for counseling alcoholic pregnant women to abort. While this move of drawing upon legislation from other fields might seem odd, it was not unusual. In other Danish clinical contexts in which I have conducted fieldwork, clinicians would not only reflect on what they personally considered good care and "the right decision" in light of guidelines for their field. They would also bring into discussions guidelines and normative frameworks from other areas of health care in an effort to broaden the perspective and reach a position on what would be the right kind of care in a particular situation. In the case of the infant of the alcoholic mother, the clinicians substituted for the infant at the margins of life not only by assisting the mother in carrying her child as long as possible, but also by thinking in terms of welfare state frameworks for who should be let into society. They placed themselves in the "we" of the welfare state, drawing upon guidelines and striving to make sense of them. Their substitution work provided an entry into the making of the welfare state at the edge of life.

In these medical rounds, an initial statement—such as the one made by the senior resident—was not a conclusive dictate. Rather, it was intended to open the conversation and generate reflections and points of views among the doctors around the table. This was what happened in this meeting. The chief neonatologist, who had long experience in the field and was highly respected, pointed out that if the child survived despite not receiving active treatment, his or her condition would be worse than if active treatment had been provided. The neonatologist argued for either palliative care or wholehearted active treatment. Another resident physician intervened. "In a way, the system has already decided to let this child live," she said, thereby expressing the idea that the social authorities bore some responsibility for the woman's not terminating her pregnancy, since both formal regulation and the social workers involved had not helped her achieve the abortion she wanted. They had not honored their part of the contract between the citizen and state institutions by ending the life of the fetus earlier.

This discussion of a premature infant expected to be born with fetal alcohol syndrome illustrates what I observed many times: there is no way to avoid selection, and the doctors take this responsibility and negotiate it among themselves before and along with approaching the parents. In the case of this infant, tentative questions of viability were raised when it became clear to the clinicians that the child would need a foster family. In an interview that Laura Emdal Navne (one of my graduate students) and I conducted with the new head of the clinic, Dr. Hans, a few years later, he said,

> A child only has a life if it has a family. That means you may save a child's life, but if the family can't handle that child, then what kind of life does this child get? Even though we live in a welfare state in Denmark, I have to say that what this society has to offer a parentless child is not good enough. Some are happy to get a foster family and actually live a family life, but many of these children end up moving between one public institution and another because the foster parents can't handle them. That is in no way a good life compared to the life in a nuclear family. This means that if the parents are strongly against having a child with severe disabilities (*tilstrækkelig meget imod, at et barn lever med svært handicap*) then that is in itself a sufficient argument. . . . Well then there have to be damn good reasons to fight for that child's survival.[9]

It was difficult to believe that the child expected to be born with fetal alcohol syndrome would have the "good life" secured by growing up in a family that Dr. Hans talked about. Moreover, as the mother had wanted an abortion, the "damn good reasons" were not present at first sight. To sum up, two things happened at the medical round. First, the chief neonatologist pointed out that the child might survive even without active care. Second, the resident physician emphasized the failed obligations of the social authorities, thus extending the child's history back to the seventeenth week of pregnancy and placing the child in a reciprocal relationship with the welfare state. In highlighting this past, the conversation underlined that by failing to provide an abortion at seventeen weeks as the mother desired, the state provided the fetus with a future—a life that began because the state had allowed it to live. The doctors saw themselves as an extension of the system that had let the child live, which made them responsible for it. As they talked about these failed obligations of the social authorities, they were already moving the unborn infant across the border of viability and turning it into a biographical life. This movement from an initial no to treatment to the final yes reflected the clinic's deep commitment to contribute to the health and survival of vulnerable infants and simultaneously secure a fair use of public funds by optimizing infant health as much as possible: active treatment would provide better chances for this child than nonactive treatment.

Staff members' conversations with Hannah's father and the medical round about the child expected to be born with fetal alcohol syndrome may seem to have little to do with the piglets in the laboratory. Nevertheless, kinship and the welfare state also play a central role in configuring the lives of the piglets and in reaching a decision about continuing or ending those lives. First, in the Newborn Pig Facility, the parent-offspring relationship, which turns Hannah into a biographical life worth fighting for, is absent. On the first day of the study, the removal of the piglets from the mother sow and their emplacement in the laboratory support the understanding of the piglets as nonsentient biological lives that need to get "up and running" as research tools. By juxtaposing the laboratory and the clinical practices, we see that the work of making the piglet into a nongrievable biological life implies not acknowledging kinship relations. In the first part of the medical round, when the senior resident suggests abstaining from active treatment, the infant's uncertain viability and its absence of socially stable kinship relations in some ways come to resemble the relations of the research piglet: the infant expected to be born with fetal alcohol syndrome appears as a nongrievable biological life divorced from social and moral relations. Juxtaposing life beginnings in the NICU and the Newborn Pig Facility clearly shows that the work of constituting a grievable biographical life involves embedding the neonate in a family. As we saw in chapter 2, this is also the case in the Newborn Pig Facility—where kinning between piglets and researchers makes the piglets appear as grievable biographical lives if only for brief moments of time. This means that the distinction between biology and biography not only marks a distinction between ontological categories like human and animal, but is present within them (Oliver 2007).

Second, the relationship to the welfare state plays a role in both settings, although in different ways. In the case of the infant of the alcoholic mother, the doctors give priority to the reciprocal relationship between citizen and state (i.e., social workers have failed to meet their obligations toward mother and child), thus moving this child across the border of viability and including it in the welfare state collectivity. We might see this as an example of kinning with the state, as the mother's inability to care for herself or the fetus turns the state into kin responsible for keeping the infant alive. The social authorities failed to intervene earlier (i.e., to provide an abortion) and thus unintentionally came to substitute for the child, which turned the state into a co-parent. Thus, in spite of the absence of a family and despite the likelihood that the infant will become an economic burden to the welfare state, the clinicians remained reluctant to abstain from active treatment. In their negotiations, two imagined welfare states compete: the cost-effective welfare state that reduces the costs of burdensome lives ("this infant . . . shall not be given active treatment," as the senior resident puts it) and the benevolent welfare state that is ready to care for all citizens ("the system has already decided to let this child live," as another resident says). In their arguments for withholding care and for providing active treatment, the clinicians invoke the responsibility of the welfare state, interpret regulations and specific practices, and treat the welfare state as the natural ground on which they stand. Here, substitution becomes an act that protects and preserves not only the life of the child, but also the welfare state. In most cases I observed, the clinicians' preference for the benevolent welfare state and what they saw as a moral imperative to sustain and care for human life propelled the child into the human collective.

The same is true in the Newborn Pig Facility, where the potential to create a particular kind of relationship with the welfare state also happens to be crucial to life-and-death decision making. Yet in this setting, the moral challenge is different. Here, the researchers never lose sight of the instrumental role of the pig. Piglets are unambiguously treated as a resource to feed into the future viability of newborn infants, including fragile neonates with alcoholic parents. If the researchers encounter a pig that cannot be turned into societal benefit, it will be put down without further ado, as we saw in the "hopeless" situation of the piglet breathing only every second minute (see the introduction). In both the Newborn Pig Facility and the human NICU, the professionals balance a concern for the welfare state collectivity with a concern for the individual neonate, yet the two concerns have different weight in the two contexts. In the animal facility, the researchers are ready to tolerate a certain amount of suffering on the part of the individual pig as long as there is a chance that its suffering may be turned into medical knowledge that will benefit the welfare state collectivity. In the NICU, the clinicians are ready to tolerate a certain amount of suffering on the part of the individual infant in the present and future and its economic burden on the welfare state as long as the infant is wanted by its parents and can be saved and placed in a reciprocal relationship with the welfare state.

In both sites, the Danish values that guide decision making embody a readiness among professionals far from the state administration to represent the welfare state and imagine and assess the character and potential of the reciprocal relationship between the welfare state and the liminal life in their care. While the kin relations of some (human) precarious neonates turn them into unquestionable biographical lives and make them become human citizens considered able to stand in a reciprocal relationship with the welfare state, the absence of kinship for other (pig) neonates turn them into nongrievable biological lives to become resources of the welfare state. Nevertheless, stepping closer to these processes, we see the instability of these categories. In the following section, I explore how not only social relations but also temporal imaginaries are crucial to the configurations of biological life, biographical life, and their porosity.

TIME: IMAGINING THE FUTURE

A few days after the medical rounds at which the infant of the alcoholic woman was discussed, she gave birth to a girl named Kathryn. The physician responsible for the baby's care told me that at birth she looked fine and was able to breathe without respiratory assistance. Given Kathryn's maturity at birth, the physicians suspected that her gestational age was higher than initially estimated in the first medical round. The fact that Kathryn breathed spontaneously removed any doubt from the professionals. In my conversation with the physician after her birth, the infant with an alcoholic mother had become a rather uncomplicated case. All the uncertainties and considerations in the doctors' initial discussions had vanished.

Kathryn's obvious viability forged a natural entry for her into life. In this situation, no clinician would find it ethically acceptable to question continuous treatment. Kathryn appeared as uncontested biographical life bearing hope and potentiality.[10] This indeterminacy also came to the fore in Hannah's father's reasoning about giving her a chance—a phrase commonly used when parents and clinicians decided to continue treatment. Other common phrases when a child was moved off the ventilator were "making it choose itself" and "letting it sail with its own sails." These phrases express a strong belief in the potentiality of newborn life (undetermined chances) and an inclination to endow the infant with agency and moral capabilities (being able to choose) in shaping its future.

In his exploration of the ways in which fiction is oriented toward endings, the literary theorist Frank Kermode draws a distinction between two Greek temporal concepts, *kairos* and *chronos*. The former refers to the moments in which time is experienced as charged with meaning and significance, whereas the latter refers to the mere successiveness of time passing, as in "one damn thing after the other" (Kermode 2000, 47). When Kathryn arrived and breathed by herself, her visible life potential provided her with a temporal horizon of *kairos*. She instantly gained what the clinicians referred to as "prospects" (*udsigt*). Among clinicians, intubation and complicated and painful operations established *kairos* as long as there was a hope that these interventions would make possible an open-ended temporality that went beyond the weeks and months of hospital care.

So what does it mean to have prospects and be placed in an open-ended perspective? In conversations with Laura and myself, Dr. Hans used a particular phrase: he needed, he said, "to imagine that the child would be able to come back to him in the future and say thank you." [11] With this phrase, he let us know that in daily care he substituted for the child by trying to stand in its place and see if he could envision a future in which his treatment would have led to the child's living a life she or he felt was worth living—which implied gaining the mental and physical capacity to move in an open space (come back) and communicate in a positive way (say thank you). Having prospects entailed the anticipation of gaining capacities of agency and reflection that would enable some kind of life that seemed meaningful to the child itself.

A visible sign of infants coming back and saying thank you was the posters made by parents of discharged children that decorated the entryway of the NICU. These posters included photos and short notes depicting the stories of the children and the trajectory of their treatments. The posters all started with the gestational day and weight of the child and continued with what had happened during his or her time in the hospital—in particular, the critical and joyful events. They ended by showing that the child, in alliance with experts, had crossed the border, entered the home, and begun a normal life with his or her parents. The posters in the NICU placed the infants in an open temporality and in affective relations that provided a home for them outside the clinic.

In most cases when clinicians cared for critically ill infants, standing by the incubator through the whole night, regulating the oxygen saturation, and constantly keeping an eye on the skin color of the infant, coming back and saying thank you was not necessarily a future that was hard to imagine. In some situations, however, clinicians' efforts to compensate for a child's malfunctioning organs (the sociomaterial component of substitution) and step into the situation of the child (the moral and affective component of substitution) made them doubt the child's prospects. Tobias was such a case.[12] He was born at thirty weeks gestation with a rare and fatal heart defect. After his birth, scans were conducted and discussed among the heart specialists. An operation was considered, although the physicians were not too optimistic that he would survive it. He was baptized in the clinic, and cards with messages such as "Congratulations from Grandma and Bobby" were placed on the small table next to him. Among the clinicians, his case was not simply a standard heart problem. Substituting for him entailed medically sustaining his body with advanced technology along with continually discussing, interpreting, and reinterpreting his scans and clinical appearance and stepping into his and his parents' positions and imagining their future. Everyone around him participated in assessing his prospects and hope of recovery.

However, at the morning conference on the third day of Tobias's life, the pediatric cardiologist reported that after having seen the newest scans, the team of surgeons considered the operation futile. He said: "How many children will get out [of the hospital] and live a normal life after five months in intensive care? It looks as if [an operation] will lead to the wrong outcome. What we are talking about is a baby in intensive care with an open sternum and after all it will lead to an unhappy ending." In other words, even with surgery, Tobias would die in the near future. In her powerful work on the temporal organization of death in American hospitals, Sharon Kaufman describes the crucial shift occurring in end-of-life care from trying to stabilize a patient to acknowledging that he or she is dying. This shift creates an impetus to "move things along" (2005, 95) and facilitate death through specific decisions and actions (99). In the case of Tobias, the morning conference demonstrated this shift and moved Tobias into the category of dying. How did this happen?

The different staff members who had taken care of Tobias and his parents had expected that he would have surgery and were sorry and upset about the decision not to operate. Yet given the newest scans, they all acknowledged and supported that decision. They all envisioned that his present suffering would continue until death, and thus his life was experienced as successive time, endless *chronos*. To them, withdrawing treatment became the most benevolent act, which transformed the mere successiveness of time passing into *kairos*, "a point in time filled with significance, charged with meaning derived from its relation to the end" (Kermode 2000, 47). After hearing the clinicians' recommendation not to operate, Tobias's mother said, "You cannot do anything good for Tobias?" The heart surgeon replied that they could do something good. "We think that the best we can do for him is not to operate," he said. In this conversation, withdrawing treatment "harmonize[d] origin and end" (Kermode 2000, 48) and established a kind of fulfillment for Tobias, his parents, and the staff. The absence of a future life for him without pain and in a proper home shaped the deliberations about his viability. The moralizing language of the surgeon and Tobias's mother ("doing good") shows their efforts to constitute him as biography and grievable life even though he did not have prospects. They extended his biographical life beyond death.

In my conversation with the heart physician later that day, he described to me all the risks of the possible operation and also touched on the situation of Tobias's parents, commenting that "most parents fall apart as they spend their lives in the hospital for several months [without the prospect of bringing their baby home]." In contrast to Kathryn's parents, Tobias's had wanted their child from the very beginning. His mother was finishing medical school, and his father had finished his training and had a job. It was not the lack of parenting abilities that led the clinicians to question Tobias's viability, but the prospect of a painful period in the hospital for both baby and parents that was anticipated to end with Tobias's death. In this way, the attention to stable and happy family lives— reflected in Danish reproductive policies—loomed in the background of the fraught process of making decisions about Tobias. His case shows that investments in saving preterm infants coexist with the possibility of discontinuing treatment if clinicians and parents do not see some kind of *kairos* for the child. As one neonatologist put it, "With premature infants, it is not that difficult to let go because the start button has not yet been pressed."[13] His metaphor conveys premature life as existing at the margins not only of life but also of time and society. There is a space for decision making when a biography has not yet begun, or when life's worth has not become fully intrinsic, so to speak.

To end my analysis of temporal imaginaries in practices of substitution, I return to the Newborn Pig Facility. Here, the NICU infants constituted the piglets' origin as well as their prospects of a meaningful future. In taking care of the piglets, the researchers did not expect the piglets to come back and say thank you. In this setting, the stop button of substitution was kill day. Death paved the way for an indeterminate future and placed the piglets in the temporal order of aevum (between worldly time and eternity), as we saw in chapter 2. Despite all the differences between the two settings, the tension between *chronos* (successive time) and *kairos* (time charged with meaning) is present in both sites. In the Newborn Pig Facility, when researchers faced piglets that were suffering more than what the researchers considered to be ethically acceptable, they strove to make a decision that would make the life and death of the piglet meaningful by connecting it to the future of society, as described in the case of piglet Huxley in chapter 2. However, there was always a risk that this goal could not be reached. At some point in their work, most researchers had experienced prolonged piglet suffering and found that piglets died by themselves, in which case the life of the piglet and the working lives of the researchers came to belong to the temporal order of *chronos*—with endless suffering and care work until death. Likewise, we may see the clinicians' decision not to operate on Tobias as a way to avoid a situation of endless suffering and institutional care until death.

In the NICU and the Newborn Pig Facility, suffering provided the neonate with sentience, a point of view, and agency. Suffering contributed to making neonates appear as biographical lives and prompted a decision about either continuing or ending treatment. If there was a prospect for a good future life—either in the form of a future life without suffering for the infant or in the form of a valuable sample for the research team—suffering was more easily tolerated. In both settings, temporal imaginaries came to constitute ethical frameworks in life-and death-making practices, highlighting the efforts that go into producing *kairos* (not just *chronos*) for liminal lives as a hallmark of care across different sites in Denmark.

SPACE: TRACING LIVES THROUGH DEATH

Ethnographies about respiratory treatment and organ donation at the end of life reveal the many ambiguities related to human personhood when bodies are sustained by intensive treatment in high-tech hospital settings. In these situations, the common Euro-American notion that death is the end of human personhood raises questions about the status of the human when his or her body breathes but no brain function is detectable (Jensen 2016; Kaufman 2005; Lock 2002). In the NICU, death did not act as a hard border that immediately turned biographical life into neutral biological life or put an end to the body's belonging in family and society. Rather, the infant as biographical life persisted beyond death. In this section, I trace the spatial arrangements through which life is constituted as biology and biography. While my focus is on practices in the NICU, I let practices in the Newborn Pig Facility act as a prism to expose the implicit relationship between human and pig that is involved in caring for and storing dead bodies.

Caroline, who was born in week twenty-six, had a twin sister, Anna, who died at birth. Some weeks after Anna's burial, the following conversation about the burial plot took place between the twins' mother and the nurse as they stood next to Caroline's incubator.

MOTHER: The stone arrived yesterday.
NURSE: What does it say?
MOTHER: It says Anna and shows a star with her date of birth and a cross with her date of death. . . . She had to have her own place. We want to go out there with Caroline. It will be easier for her to understand [that she has a dead twin sister] when Anna has her own place and does not rest among all the others.

To Caroline's mother, not resting "among all the others" provided her dead daughter with a place that was not public and anonymous, but personal and home-like. The personal grave marked a place of belonging for the child buried there and created a space for the family to keep the memory and the story of her alive. In this conversation, the work of biography was directed not only at the living Caroline in the incubator, but also at her dead sibling, Anna. By providing Anna with her own place outside medical institutions, her singularity was maintained, as was the living girl's continued kinship with her sister. A little later in the conversation, the mother said: "You know, the burial plot—I would have liked to have had it in Jylland [the western part of Denmark, several hours' drive from the hospital in Copenhagen]. That was a bit hard to accept in the beginning."

Although the chosen burial plot was very close to where the mother and father of Anna lived, the mother's wish for a plot on the same soil where she had grown up illustrates the connections between kinship and geographical location in constituting the child as biography. In Anna's case, the personal burial plot played a role in avoiding the identity of nongrievable biological life.

Some weeks after this incident, the spatial component in constituting life as biology or biography became even more visible to me. In the morning conference, the weekend team reported that a girl born at term had died twenty-four hours after birth. From the moment of birth, she had hovered between life and death and was put in the heart-and-lung machine, which sustains the body in life even when the heart and lungs shut down and thus represents the ultimate sociomaterial substitution. When the girl suffered a massive bleeding in the brain, the doctors and her parents were confronted with troubling moral questions about how far to continue her treatment—what I have referred to as the affective and moral component of substitution—and in the end they decided not to provide further treatment. Through the day, I followed the nurse responsible for the parents and the dead girl. As we entered their room, the parents stood weeping next to the small hospital bassinet that contained their child. A drawing by the couple's three-year-old son and a photo of the parents decorated the crib. The parents' grief was present in every item in the room. Standing next to them, the nurse said, "She looks peaceful." "Yes," the father answered tearfully, "she is in a better state now than when she was downstairs [in intensive care], when she was pricked constantly and tugged. . . . We have told her all the things to be said. We have kissed and hugged her." Encountering their grief as they bowed over their perfectly normal looking, but dead, child, I felt a lump in my throat. I realized that I did not have such feelings when handling dead piglet bodies. Why did I take for granted that the infant was grievable, but the pigs were not?

"Are you ready for her to be moved away?" the nurse asked. The parents nodded. The nurse and I had come to move the girl from the room of the parents, as she needed to be refrigerated until she was moved to the chapel. The nurse asked the parents if they had written a letter to the girl. With tears running down her cheeks, the mother replied that they had not yet done so. The nurse kept assuring the parents that even though we would take the girl with us, she would not be far away, and they could always ask to see her again. When the nurse and I said goodbye to the parents and left the room, the nurse made sure that the baby blanket covered the face of the girl so it was not visible as we wheeled the bassinet down the hall. We were silent. It simply did not feel right to comment on the child or the parents in grief or begin a more ordinary conversation. To me, our silence was not only a way of taking in the tragic and heartbreaking situation of the parents, but also a way of respecting their grief and the dead child in front of us.

The nurse planned to put the dead body in the fridge of the maternity ward. This fridge was where the bodies of infants aborted late in pregnancy, placentas,

and the occasional dead child were stored before they were moved to other destinations—be it the chapel, the dissection table, the medical waste container, or
research laboratories. However, the nurse told me, she found it improper to
bring the dead child through the maternity ward where we might encounter
other mothers. Before entering, she wanted to make sure that she would be able
to bring the child directly to the fridge. Just outside the ward, she found an
empty office. She grabbed a big post-it note, wrote "*mors*"—the Latin word for
death—on it, and put the note on the child's blanket. In that way, other health
professionals who might have entered the office during the few minutes we were
gone would know that the bassinet contained a dead child. Although the door to
the office was open when we arrived, the nurse closed it to discourage people
from entering. The two of us went to the maternity ward, where the nurse asked
a midwife, "Do you have space in the fridge for a child that is *mors*?" The midwife
said yes, and we walked the short distance to the "skyllerum," a storage room for
supplies and medical waste, where the nurse opened a big steel cupboard whose
size and design were quite similar to an ordinary fridge. As soon as the nurse had
made sure that there was space for the bassinet with the girl, we returned to the
office. We threw out the post-it note and wheeled the girl to the storage room in
the maternity ward. On the top shelves of the fridge were trays with baby blan-
kets. On top of each blanket was a stack of papers, which looked like medical
journals. The nurse informed me that these were the bodies of two other much
smaller children, probably late abortions. Some placentas were also in the fridge.
The nurse lifted the bassinet from its base, but had trouble getting it into the
fridge. "I know there is room for a bassinet. I have done it before," she commented. By placing the bassinet at a slight angle, she eventually succeeded in
squeezing it on the bottom shelf.

The journey from the parents' room to the fridge in the "skyllerum" transformed the girl's identity from biographical life to biological life through spatial
arrangements. In the room with the parents, the girl was thoroughly defined by
her kin relations, as we also saw in the case of Emily. The parents' grief, their
attachment to her, their decorations on her bassinet, and the nurse's and the
father's statements about peace constituted the girl as grievable biographical life
placed in relationships and deserving care in another way than a biological body
"pricked and tugged" in the ICU. When we left their room, the nurse and I
upheld this grievable, biographical life situated in social relations by treating the
girl's death as private, keeping silent and invisibilizing her body. The nurse's
efforts to cover the child's body and keep it at a safe distance from the activities
of bringing new babies into life in the maternity ward upheld the hospital as an
institution engaged in life, not death, and treated death as a contradiction to life.
This well-known life imperative supported the understanding of human life as
holding an open future, thus indirectly placing the girl in the category of human
biographical life.

In the maternity ward and the NICU, every hospital routine was directed toward bringing infants into life with the expectation that they would eventually live at home with their parents. In this setting, there was certainly no kill day, and there was no loud talk about death and dissection—although a small minority of children did die, and some of them were even dissected and used for research. The contrast with the Newborn Pig Facility was illuminating. In the facility, there was no possibility of a pig's leaving the scientific institution, either alive or dead. The integration of laboratory life and the life of the singular piglet helped constitute the piglet as plain biological nongrievable life. In other words, constituting piglets as a resource for human infants was enabled by housing piglets in a state institution and linking viable infants to a home and a territory outside such institutions.

The Latin word *mors* on the post-it note and in the conversation with the midwife loosened the girl from her social relationships. This word, which is widely used in the medical field, denotes death as a biological phenomenon and thus separated the girl from her grieving parents and connected her to medical practices and the medical institution.[14] As she was put in the fridge next to "all the others," she moved closer to biological life. The fridge is a container, a space for storage. A subject (the nurse) moves an object (the girl) into storage.[15] However, the girl whose body was placed in the fridge just below aborted fetuses and placentas was not cut up and distributed into research samples, as was the case with the pigs. Rather, the girl kept her bodily integrity, signaling intrinsic worth—similar to Anna's getting her own place at the cemetery. Moreover, the nurse told the girl's parents that they could see her again if they wanted. Although containing her in the fridge moved her closer to biological life, she continued to be recognized as a grievable biographical life and kept her baby blanket, which signified a personal space.

What does this juxtaposition of spatial arrangements of dead bodies in lab and clinic teach us? It shows that life as grievable biography is enacted by treating death as located in and affecting social relations and as constituting the unplanned exception. In contrast, life as biology is enacted by treating death as nongrievable and as a planned and calculated event integrated with the scientific institution. Moreover, the tension between biographical and biological life, or grievable and nongrievable life, that appears in both the NICU and the Newborn Pig Facility reveals how borders between these two configurations are in no way self-evident. The situations of Julie with the anesthetized piglet in her arms and the nurse and me squeezing the dead girl onto the shelf in the fridge expose how both piglets and infants may vacillate between biological and biographical life, as these configurations are mobile and multiple. Drawing bodies into dimensions of biographical life or dimensions of nonpersonal biology is a social, temporal, and spatial achievement.

RESOURCE DISCUSSIONS IN THE NICU

The cases of Emily, Hannah, Kathryn, and Tobias spell out how care for infants on the verge of life is not necessarily experienced as antithetical to suffering. Continued care may produce suffering, which is considered acceptable if that suffering ultimately moves the infant toward a life that is meaningful—in other words, a life which is fulfilling for the child itself and for which the child can come back and say thanks, a life which will contribute to a well-functioning family, and a life enabling reciprocal relationship between citizen and state. Yet a focus on these reciprocal obligations, particularly as a reason for giving or withholding care, might seem at odds with the principles of the egalitarian welfare state. What kinds of moral reasoning are involved in withholding care in a country in which every citizen is entitled not only to health care in an emergency but also to lifelong continuous universal health services and social support, and in which all citizens are considered equal? Why would medical professionals in an affluent country like Denmark think it natural to initiate discussions about abstaining from treatment or withdrawing treatment in certain critical cases? To answer these questions, I first turn to the presence of economic prioritizations and notions of societal sustainability in resource discussions among doctors in the NICU. I then turn to Danish reproductive health policies since the 1930s and provide a historical perspective on the coexistence of practices of selection and care in welfare state policies of providing equal support and life prospects for every citizen.

In the NICU, when infants were hovering between life and death, making decisions about the initiation or continuation of treatment was one of the hardest things clinicians had to do. The cases of Cheung (discussed in the introduction) and of Kathryn, Emily, Tobias, and Hannah (discussed in this chapter) show that these discussions involved "moral wrestling" (Sharp 2019, 8) in which there was no simple answer to the question "what is a life worth living?" Despite the lack of such an answer, what guided clinical decision making was the inclusionary norm of putting the child in a reciprocal relationship to his or her family and the welfare state within an open-ended temporal frame. Yet explicit deliberations about resources did enter discussions among clinicians in the very rare cases where parents resisted the clinicians' recommendations to withdraw treatment. In one such case,[16] the clinicians considered continued treatment futile, yet the parents were not willing to withdraw treatment. They insisted on continued treatment and clung to the hope that a miracle might happen and that death was not the only possible future for their child. Commenting on this case, Dr. Hans said: "Overall, resources are not unlimited. Shall we continue with a very care-intensive treatment, which is futile and painful for the patient?" He and his staff members did not think they should do so, as continuing treatment for such an infant would take up a space in the NICU and exclude other infants who, with care and technology, might become viable babies. Also, spending time and money on treating an infant without prospects would exhaust the staff, whose members were already working full out and doing their utmost to make other infants viable, and for whom the experience of success in creating worthy lives was essential to maintain faith in their work. Thus, in the contested cases, the doctors did not blindly follow parents' wishes for continued treatment and prolonged life. Rather, the work of substituting for infants on the fringes of life involved balancing the situation of the family and the resources of the clinic and the welfare state.

This way of placing the infant in relation to the resources of the welfare state also came to the fore in an interview with Dr. Tina. Reflecting upon the many considerations that the clinicians must take into account in life-and-death decision making, she said: "We [as medical doctors] have a societal responsibility. The children we help live should be able to fend for themselves." In another conversation, she said: "If you let a child with multiple disabilities enter society, it is very resource-intensive. I don't think so much about it in general, but we need to do it [think about it], and it is part of medical work to do so." With her latter remark, Dr. Tina was reminding herself of the moral obligation to serve society— which is part of the Hippocratic oath, as that is interpreted by the Danish medical profession. To her, paying attention to society was a way of contributing to a fair distribution of resources and thus staying in relations of solidarity with the present and future members of the welfare state collectivity.

In explaining the efforts put into saving infants at the margins of life, a nurse in the NICU said, "we have many valuable infants in this clinic." With this statement, she referred to the fact that many infants—like the twins Hannah and Elisabeth—were the result of IVF treatments and thus planned and wanted by their parents, along with being costly for society. Fighting to save these children was to nurses an acknowledgment of the investments made by the state, which may have subsidized the IVF treatments, and the work performed by their colleagues in fertility clinics. The point is not that the nurses calculated the monetary cost of an IVF infant. Rather, in describing the moral dilemmas of saving infants at the margins of life, they considered both state investments and parents' lives. As Aradhana Sharma and Akhil Gupta remind us, "rather than being an outward reflection of a coherent and bounded state 'core' [everyday practices in state institutions], actually constitute that very core" (2006, 13). Dr. Tina's articulation of her obligation to serve society and the nurse's reference to "valuable infants" connected welfare state finances to their own working lives, thus producing and enacting the welfare state in the daily routines of treating infants.

Clinicians did not make explicit calculations of the cost of a child's present and future treatments. However, the notions that state resources had to be shared, and thus prioritized, and that every citizen had to contribute to the common good, not just receive services, were always present. In a conversation over lunch one day, one of the physicians commented, "Sometimes I wonder if it is at all in the interest of society that we work so hard to save these children who might never get an education or get a proper job." Substituting for children on the verge of life created ambivalence about how to take account of (and connect the life of the child to) the life of the welfare state. When clinicians discussed an infant's prospects, none of them thought it right to save a child they considered destined to become a resident in an institution. This view reflected both Dr. Hans's concern about the child's quality of life ("[life in an institution] is in no way a good life compared to a life in a nuclear family") and Dr. Tina's concern about welfare state resources ("the children we help live should be able to fend for themselves"). Thereby the doctors were not only taking into account the situation of the family, when infants were at the margins of life and their entry into society contested. The doctors also included in their deliberations the child's potential to enter relationships with the welfare state, and hence, they saw the child as a resource for both the family and the welfare state collectivity. Let me be clear: clinicians did not think of contributions in solely economic terms. They were very aware that a disabled child could be an enormous contribution to his or her parents and siblings, as well as to the community, yet they did not take those contributions for granted. Rather, in their discussion, the doctors considered whether it was likely that this particular child and family would experience a good and productive quality of life. The first part of the clinical discussion about the alcoholic mother also reflected this perspective: saving a child needs to make sense in terms of the family and the welfare state.

The clinicians' deliberations about societal resources resonate with public discourse in Denmark. In news reporting on political discussions, in conversations among friends or colleagues, and at meetings at the local school or in the many associations Danes are part of, the prioritization of public resources (i.e., how to spend taxpayers' money on different groups of citizens and make ends meet) is a common theme of discussion. To Danes, questions about prioritization do not belong simply to economics and the domain of state finance. They are moral questions because they concern what society to build and live in, as well as which citizens to include in Danish society, which has the goals of universal access to welfare services and a high level of equality among residents. Central to Danish prioritization discussions is a strong idea of scarcity (Spalletta 2021), which has intensified with neoliberal incursions, for instance, in the form of performance-based management in hospitals and stricter conditions for citizens requesting welfare benefits. At the time of my fieldwork in the NICU, Danish prioritization discussions were mostly about benefits for social groups (for example, providing early pensions for long-term workers, stipends for students, and benefits for the unemployed). When it came to health care, politicians usually refrained from making explicit statements on which treatments were unaffordable and instead upheld the ideal that every citizen has intrinsic worth and should be cared for.

However, as elsewhere in the Danish health services, in the NICU, the financial implications of providing treatment were inevitable and NICU staff members were confronted with making decisions about individuals.[17] Resource management included ensuring that some resource-demanding infants did not take attention away from other infants with greater needs and retaining staff members by providing working conditions in which they were able to see their work as meaningful—thereby facilitating the future availability of human resources for the welfare state. Every treatment had a price known to staff members, the clinic had a budget to meet, there were prices on each item in the medicine room of the clinic, and only the most premature infants were allowed to be fed the costly human donor milk. Even so, the clinicians did not consider it morally acceptable to bring up the issue of resource management when talking to the parents. Why not?

Reflecting on this, Dr. Hans said to Laura and me: "I think that it is unethical [to mention the issue of money to the parents]. . . . They are in the deepest imaginable crisis in their lives. . . . Money is of no relevance in comparison to life and death. How can the two of them [money and life or death] come together?" While these two could not be separated in the daily management of the clinic and prioritizing lives, the clinicians separated issues of money and life when talking to the parents. Thus, the inescapable question of which lives to treat, given limited societal resources, constituted a specific geography—a "careography" (Navne and Svendsen 2018)—that separated the spaces in which resource questions could be known and discussed (the daily rounds and interviews with anthropologists) from the spaces in which resource questions were unknown (conversations with parents).[18] For the clinicians, unknowing resource issues in conversations with parents was a way of caring for the parents in their grief and maintaining a high degree of empathy and understanding in relationships with them.

The absence of resource prioritizations in conversations with parents illuminates a difference in money talk between the Newborn Pig Facility and the NICU. In the facility, the researchers' articulations of a connection between economic value and pig life (as researchers described in chapter 2, "a euthanized piglet costs a piglet at the other end") constitutes the pig as a neutral biological life valuable as a resource for humans. In the NICU, the clinicians avoided mentioning the calculability of life in front of the parents and thus underlined the human infant as noncalculable—that is, as a grievable biographical life with intrinsic worth. Hence, by not exposing the inescapable prioritizations present in daily clinical practice, the clinicians separated the value of money from the value of human life, while not losing sight of the infant standing in a reciprocal resource relationship to the welfare state. Like the researchers, who performed virtuous acts of caring for the vulnerable piglets and the big picture of improving health for vulnerable infants, the clinicians constantly strove to find the right balance between, on the one hand, helping parents through the grieving process and returning to everyday life outside the NICU and, on the other hand, the big picture of securing a fair use of resources.

SELECTIVE REPRODUCTIVE POLITICS IN DENMARK

To better understand this attention to the big picture, I turn now to Danish reproductive health politics since the 1930s, focusing on eugenics in the beginning of the twentieth century and prenatal diagnostics in the 1970s and at the beginning of the twenty-first century. By turning to the history of selective reproductive politics in Denmark, I aim to show that the orientation toward collective concerns that comes to the fore in life-and-death decisions in the NICU has strong historical roots. The Danish history of human reproductive selection helps demonstrate how an orientation toward including equal human lives within a welfare state collectivity goes hand in hand with excluding lives from this collectivity.

In the 1930s, a large group of social reforms was introduced in Denmark and laid the ground for the country's welfare state. With these reforms, the state secured access to health care for all citizens and support in case of accidents, sickness, and unemployment. In the following decades, the reforms were extended, culminating in 1956 with a pension reform that provided all Danish citizens with a public pension independent of their income. These reforms not only demonstrated lawmakers' willingness to stand up for precarious citizens by replacing absent income with social benefits. They also established a contract between state and people that is characteristic of all Nordic welfare societies: the strong and benevolent state facilitates the development of an emancipated and autonomous individual, who is liberated from dependence on charities and families (Trägårdh 2002).

However, a closer look at the social reforms from the 1930s shows that in return for benefits, a certain behavior was required of citizens. In exchange for social security, the individual citizen was expected to behave responsibly in social matters, including reproduction. As it turned out, not all citizens were judged capable of fulfilling this contract. In parliamentary discussions of the proposed social reforms, a central issue was how to distinguish the deserving poor (*værdigt trængende*) from the undeserving poor (*uværdigt trængende*).[19] The deserving poor were healthy and responsible workers who were considered to be victims of hard times. The small group of the undeserving poor belonged to the "unfit" (*undermålerne*), as they were called—people who, despite economic assistance, were rarely able to improve their situation. When it came to reproduction, it was expected that the children of the undeserving poor would inherit their poor mental and social qualities, and thus the reproduction of the undeserving poor should be strictly controlled (Petersen, Petersen, and Christiansen 2013).

Karl Kristian Steincke became minister of justice in a newly elected Social Democratic government in 1924. In a major work on the Danish welfare system, he developed the basic arguments for the social and economic reforms of the 1930s (Steincke 1920). Steincke wanted to establish a morally and economically sustainable society. By the 1930s, the small minority of the unfit was seen not only as an economic burden in the present, but also as a growing threat to the future sustainability of society due to the combination of their problematic hereditary qualities and reckless reproductive behavior. Steincke articulated the concern that the quality of the population would decline due to the fact that the valuable parts of the population would give birth to too few individuals or immigrate to America, while the less valuable parts of the population would stay in Denmark and give birth to too many low-quality individuals—with people in both groups behaving in a shortsighted manner. They were thinking only of their own convenience and not about the greater social collectivity. This called for reforms. In 1929, a test act tried out a eugenic practice by offering voluntary sterilization to the unfit as well as to mentally normal citizens at risk of transmitting hereditary defects to their offspring. From this test act, a comprehensive set of social technologies was developed in the form of a group of laws that regulated the reproduction of some groups of Danes. In 1934, a law about the compulsory internment and sterilization of the so-called feebleminded (i.e., people with cognitive impairments or learning difficulties and those with psychiatric problems) was introduced, and in 1935, a law about voluntary and compulsory sterilization and castration was approved by the Danish Parliament. These laws provided the legal ground for sterilization of the feebleminded and others seen as socially dangerous.[20] The abortion law of 1937 allowed the "termination of pregnancy because of fear that the offspring had inherited physical and mental illnesses, psychological abnormalities, criminal tendencies or similar traits from the parents."[21] The marriage law of 1938 required permission to marry for those referred to as "feebleminded," "psychopaths," "alcoholics," and "epileptics," as well as others who from the point of view of present society and future generations were viewed as dangerous. Sterilization was a precondition for their marriages, and marriages entered into in violation of the rules could be annulled (Koch 2014, 135–142).

In proposing the first Danish eugenic law to address the issue of compulsory sterilization, Steincke said: "Every human being should have a right to the utmost fulfillment in life and if necessary, be protected and cared for. Only in one respect, society needs to be alert: as regards reproduction. . . . We treat the unfit with all kinds of care and love, but in return only forbid him to reproduce himself."[22] With this proposal, Steincke aimed, on the one hand, to care for all citizens. On the other hand, he aimed to reduce the costs of state care for the undeserving poor and their offspring and to reduce the number of reproductive crimes conducted by the "feebleminded" whose sexuality was considered "excessive" and whose fertility was described as "disgusting."[23] The eugenic laws were a way of preventing reproduction among people who, due to their heredity, were considered a moral and economic threat to the welfare state.

For the majority, the social reforms marked the beginning of a public sector that provided social security and individual freedom as part of democratic governance (Kolstrup 2011, 197–198; Petersen, Petersen, and Christiansen 2013, 121). This is the welfare state that many contemporary Danes encounter in positive ways when they receive services in different aspects of life—child care, education, health care, elder care, unemployment benefits, and pensions—that are available to everyone. For the minority, however, the reforms represented increased reproductive control and demonstrated a readiness to regulate lives considered less worthy and to determine who should remain unborn, thus never entering the welfare state collectivity (Kolstrup 2011, 232). The reforms demonstrated the great value put on moral and economic sustainability in early Danish welfare politics and the coexistence of care and selection in political interventions aimed at creating a sustainable society. I suggest seeing these reforms as practices of substitution, which contain both a sociomaterial component of standing in for precarious citizens by providing them with economic support, and an affective and moral component of stepping into the position of the person in need of substitution and imagining the future of his or her life in a wider social context. So far, I have investigated this moral and affective part of substitution in interactions among doctors, nurses, researchers, and precarious neonates in particular spaces and situations. For example, in making decisions about Cheung (see the introduction) and the infant of the alcoholic mother (see above in this chapter), clinicians stepped into the situation of the particular child and imagined his or her relationships to parents and the welfare state to reach a decision about continuing or withdrawing treatment. When it comes to policies, this affective and moral component of substitution may seem more distant, yet it is not absent. In the case of the social reforms of the 1930s, the state's practices of substituting for precarious citizens entailed taking a moral stance on who to support and which unborn lives to exclude from the collectivity.[24] Reproductive selection by intervening in the lives of potential parents (e.g., by way of sterilization) or terminating unborn life (e.g., by way of abortion) became part and parcel of sustaining a welfare state that was seen as both dependent on and obliged to protect its members. In this way, substitution practices illuminate a side of the state that is simultaneously benevolent and instrumental.

In the 1920s and 1930s, when Steincke presented eugenics as a means of securing a healthy population for future society, eugenics was already systematized in Danish pig production to achieve the highest possible economic return for commercial pig producers. This was no coincidence. Animal breeding experiments and eugenics belonged to the same "'epistemic space' of heredity" (Müller-Wille and Rheinberger 2005, 6) that was born in the late nineteenth century in Europe and the United States and developed throughout the first part of the twentieth century.[25] In the beginning of the twentieth century, experiments with animal breeding provided inspiration for developing social technologies for culling the least fit members of the human population. Although at the time the not-yet-born offspring of the unfit represented negative economic and moral value, Steincke strongly expressed the need for a heterogeneous population and explicitly rejected eugenics that would treat human beings as "dog or horse breeds" (Koch 2014, 95). He recommended "breeding out" the unfit, rather than the deliberate selection of desirable traits through reproductive choices. For these reasons, Steincke saw himself as supporting a multidirectional and open-ended potentiality of human development.

In the language of the time, the people considered unfit covered a diverse group, including the feebleminded, gypsies, the deaf, the blind, and people with other physical disabilities. In addition, alcoholics, criminals, and vagabonds were of interest to the eugenicists, even though their reproduction was never regulated. The feebleminded constituted the group of greatest concern to legislators. Before the age of genetic diagnostics, this category was to a great extent based on social indications (Koch 2014, 122–127). For example, poor school performance, unemployment in the family, alcohol abuse, wife beating, sexual promiscuity, low IQ scores, and stuttering contributed to the decision to consider a family at risk of producing feebleminded children (31–33).

The Danish eugenic legislation replaced the previous regulation of human reproduction, which was based on religious views and prohibited sterilization and abortion except where medically indicated. At the time, eugenics was seen by many as a progressive movement, which grounded reproductive politics in scientific facts and paved the way for individual choice in reproductive matters. The legislation was supported by people with a broad spectrum of political views. With the test act of 1929, Denmark, not Germany,[26] became the first European nation to introduce eugenic legislation that allowed for voluntary sterilization and castration. In contrast to the eugenic legislation that appeared in Germany in the 1930s, the Danish legislation passed between 1929 and 1938 was not based on a racial ideology (where Jews, e.g., were considered undesirable due to their ancestry). Nevertheless, what Denmark shared with the eugenics movement elsewhere in Europe was a preoccupation with the characteristics of the population. Steincke and his contemporaries saw the so-called healthy and productive parts of the population as an important, yet endangered, resource on which future welfare depended.[27]

In sum, the social reforms, including the eugenic reforms from 1934 and 1935 that introduced compulsory sterilization in Denmark, illustrate a logic in which the state provides benefits and care for millions of people and aims at securing healthy children for the future. For this to happen, Steincke calculated that thousands of other people had to pay with their reproductive freedom. Some children would never be conceived, and some people would never become parents. Likewise, we might say, the research piglets pay with their lives to sustain the human collective. The continuities between pig breeding and human reproductive politics and between past and present reproductive politics do not concern the governmental means used to steer reproduction. Pig breeding is certainly a world apart from the policy on compulsory sterilization, and the policy on compulsory sterilization is certainly a world apart from today's policy of informing pregnant women with alcohol problems about the possibility of abortion. The continuity I see concerns the orientation toward the collectivity and its sustainability. In both the eugenic laws and today's reproductive politics, well-functioning families are considered crucial building blocks for societal sustainability. When the Danish fertility law emphasizes parental abilities, and when Dr. Hans claims that "a child only has a life if it has a family," they echo the emphasis put on social indications in the eugenic past. In the past, evaluating the worth of potential offspring was based partly on the social situation of the family. In the present, qualifications of the parents—their abilities and willingness to care for a disabled child—are brought into life-and-death decision-making processes. The child gains worth (and has the prospect of experiencing his or her own life as meaningful) by being part of and contributing to sustainable family and societal futures. Similarly, the pig's life and death become meaningful by being connected to infants and thus to societal futures. In both past and present, integral to these processes of facilitating entry to the welfare state collectivity are exclusions—of unborn offspring of the feebleminded, limp piglets, and fragile infants who do not have open-ended futures.

In the decades following World War II, eugenics as it was practiced in Germany was strongly condemned. Nevertheless, the Danish sterilization system seemed immune to this criticism, and compulsory sterilization of the unfit remained legal and continued until 1967, while sterilization of people with other diagnoses continued until 1974 (Koch 2014, 242). At that time, however, "worn-out mothers" in need of birth control were the ones who used the sterilization law of 1935 (Koch 2000, 196–208). In the same period, several new interventions were introduced to improve reproductive health. The 1940s saw the introduction of state-financed prenatal care for all pregnant women (Vallgårda 2003). In the 1950s and 1960s, state-financed vaccination programs for children were introduced. In 1973, Denmark became one of the first countries in Western Europe to legalize abortion before the twelfth week of pregnancy, a service that became publicly financed.[28] In the 1970s, advances in cell biology and chromosomal analysis brought about new possibilities for prenatal diagnostics, and in 1978 the use of amniocentesis to detect Down syndrome was introduced free of charge for women older than thirty-five. The official white paper arguing for this to become a public service said: "By preventing births of children with lifelong disabilities in need of continuous admissions to hospitals or lifelong institutionalizations, prenatal diagnostics have a great societal potential. Prenatal diagnostics potentially prevent human tragedies. In addition, when prenatal diagnostics can be employed in such a way that from a cost-benefit perspective the societal savings balance or exceed the public expenses related to prenatal diagnostics, the commission finds that the public sector will achieve a considerable advantage by giving high priority to prenatal diagnostics in health care politics in the future."[29]

The unworthiness embedded in the notion of "human tragedy" refers to a disabled life in and out of state-financed institutions. Its prevention is unambiguously framed as the responsibility of the state, a state that aims for the sustainability of public finances and thus pursues a cost-effective system of prenatal diagnostics.[30] From this perspective, unborn children with the prospect of "lifelong disabilities" face a poor life for themselves and their families and also represent a burden on the welfare state, as they are not likely to contribute to sustaining the collectivity. Substitution in the form of high-quality, universal care (including care for disabled citizens who are institutionalized for their whole lives) coexists with a readiness to terminate pregnancies based on ideals about meaningful life and an economically sustainable welfare state.[31]

Concurrently with the introduction of prenatal diagnostics in Danish public health care, new genetic and reproductive technologies raised questions about the moral status of reproductive materials (sperm, eggs, and embryos), which now could be imagined and handled separately from the sexual act of the reproducing bodies.[32] The Danish committee established to discuss the implications of assisted reproduction published a report that challenged the cost-benefit perspective in Danish reproductive politics (Danish Ministry of Interior Affairs 1984). The report warned against singling out particular humans according to a health-economic logic and emphasized that the heterogeneity of the population and the inclusion of disabled people are valuable for the welfare state.[33] In the report, "the right to be deviant" (*retten til at være afviger*) appears as something that needs to be protected, and the autonomy of the individual woman is emphasized as an important societal value. The report forcefully expresses the normative social framework that emerged after World War II, highlighting the autonomy of the individual, disconnecting the value of human life from economic value, and stressing the role of social circumstances in shaping the quality of life.

As much as life-and-death decisions in the NICU seem in line with Steincke's concern for the larger collectivity and the cost-benefit perspective of prenatal diagnostics, these decisions also show strong continuities with the growing attention through the 1970s and 1980s to the right to be deviant. In the NICU, saving disabled infants is considered highly meaningful, as long as the child is rooted in viable family relations. The discussions among clinicians provide a unique insight into how professionals in the welfare state balance care for the individual deviant child with care for sustainable families as building blocks of society.

In 2004, a new set of official Danish guidelines on prenatal diagnostics explicitly rejected the economic argument from 1978 and framed prenatal diagnosis in the neoliberal language of personal choice.[34] This did not cause an increase in parents' using their infant's "right to be deviant."[35] In the 2010s, uptake of prenatal screening and diagnostics among pregnant women was above 90 percent, and in the case of identification of a fetus with Down syndrome, 99 percent of women abort (Barrett 2016). Ethnographic studies of women receiving prenatal diagnostics document that today women consider doing so to be a natural part of being pregnant (Heinsen 2018; Schwennesen, Svendsen, and Koch 2010). When they receive a Down syndrome diagnosis for their fetus, women see abortion as the right solution because it is an opportunity given to them by the welfare state and an act that secures their continued participation in the labor market (Heinsen 2018). This illustrates that the welfare state encourages people to see a "child-to-be as a fluid, negotiable and contested entity that is potentially 'rejectable'" (88). Although substitution in the form of social support for disabled children is available, it coexists with state-financed possibilities for discarding unborn life that is diagnosed as abnormal. Although the guidelines from 2004 were explicitly distanced from eugenic thinking, their introduction of state-financed prenatal diagnosis for all women demonstrates a continuation of selective reproduction. Yet the governmental means changed from compulsion to choice.

In the beginning of the 2000s, when I entered IVF clinics to study the donation of human embryos to human embryonic stem cell research, I observed how laboratory staff members categorized embryos according to their quality, and I encountered the pragmatic attitude of couples who willingly donated embryos of low quality (so-called waste embryos) to this new research field. Only good-looking embryos were inserted in the womb of women in an effort to optimize their chances of pregnancy and having a healthy child (Svendsen 2007, 2011; Svendsen and Koch 2008). No pro-life voices were heard inside or outside the clinic, reflecting Danes' pragmatic attitudes toward unborn life. In the twenty-first century in Denmark, selective reproduction is realized through the neoliberal discourse on choice in combination with a great trust in state-run heath care that indirectly steers the population—through individual choice—toward the same preventive effects as in the 1930s and 1970s (see Schwennesen, Svendsen, and Koch 2010; Koch 2014, 247).

JUXTAPOSING HUMAN AND PIG, PAST AND PRESENT

The first two chapters of this book illuminated the daily practices of constituting pigs as human substitutes and making their life, suffering, and death contribute to human lives. This chapter has illuminated another layer of that constitution. Here, I have placed human and pig together to understand what it takes to gain value and qualify as a certain form of life. This juxtaposition may state the obvious: humans and animals are different creatures and accordingly are treated in very different ways. Thus, one could argue that it is exactly because pigs lack human rights that they are not part of society in the way that human infants are. While I do not dispute this claim, this chapter has unhinged daily practices from discursive claims about differences and paved the way for an analysis of the social, temporal, and spatial practices through which lives are differentiated. At the same time as the ethnography shows that the absence of kinship, an open future, and a home is crucial to differentiating the pig from the human and setting up boundaries between biographical and biological life, it also demonstrates that these boundaries are not stable. When is the human fetus of the alcoholic mother a nongrievable biological life? When is it a grievable biographical human life in peril? When is the piglet in Julie's arms a grievable biographical life entangled in interspecies kin relations? When is it a nongrievable biological life? Following the oscillating qualities of the configurations of biological life and biographical life exposes the borders of the human and reminds us that not every human may become a grievable biographical life, and not every pig may become a nongrievable biological life.

Anthropology has always aimed at uncovering cultural differences and been sensitive to the many different ways of being human. However, in investigating those many different ways, anthropologists have turned to their human interlocutors and described their ways of reasoning and acting. Tobias Rees refers to this way of approaching the human as a mode of cataloguing: "Who makes up people? Who creates new labels? The answer is people" (2018, 47). And he adds, "there is a somehow unchanging anthropology according to which people make up people." While my ethnography mostly stays with human actors, my movement between the Newborn Pig Facility and the human NICU nevertheless creates an uncertainty about the anthropological catalog of how humans make up humans. The practices of substitution I have uncovered show that grievable biographical (human) life is not separable from nongrievable biological (pig) life. There is a symbiopolitical relationship between the two, as the viability and homing of the child implicates the housing and killability of the piglets. Human neonate and pig neonate are "yoked" together and belong in the same litter (Haraway 2016, 110).

At the same time as this chapter has pointed to the practices that distinguish the human from the pig, my juxtapositions of human and animal sites and past and present selective reproductive politics also highlight that relationships to the Danish welfare state shape not only the life and death of infants and piglets, but also the value ascribed to them. Where a meaningful life for the research piglet is to provide good data for the welfare state in the far future, in the NICU, happy family lives and reciprocal relationships to the state in the near future are key markers for professionals who steer decision-making processes for infants on the fringes of life. If we stay on the human side, we see that in both the eugenic past, in present prenatal diagnostics, and in life-and-death decision making in the NICU, intrinsic worth does not necessarily stand in opposition to instrumental worth. Rather, the lives included in the welfare state come to hold intrinsic worth the moment they enter a family in a home and enter reciprocal moral and economic relationships with the welfare state collectivity, which is expected to last for life.

If this chapter has revealed the inclusionary norms at the heart of situating the individual infant and piglet in relationship to the welfare state collectivity, my ethnography and policy analyses have also uncovered the fact that these inclusionary norms are exclusionary. Birth not only works as a natural entry to life and society, it also constitutes a border zone for selecting who and what belongs in society. Substitution practices in this border zone reveal that egalitarianism and reciprocity as strong social values are at the center of excluding unborn lives and born piglets and infants at the margins of life. As chapter 4 shows, notions of collectivity and belonging are also involved in letting into or pushing out of society human and animal lives across geographical borders.

4 · METABOLIZING
Humans and Nonhumans in a Global Field

It is January 2017, and the NEOCOL research platform is being launched in a packed meeting room at the School of Veterinary Medicine and Animal Science at the University of Copenhagen, in the same building that houses the Newborn Pig Facility. Along one wall, seven collaborators from clinics and laboratories in China have found seats. Next to them, I recognize neonatologists from New Zealand, England, the Netherlands, and Australia whom I have met at previous meetings. Danish PhD students, postdoctoral students, and professors make up another substantial part of the group. This gathering is the culmination of the NEOMUNE research platform that began four years earlier at the colostrum collection sites on Danish dairy farms, in the intestines of research piglets in the Newborn Pig Facility downstairs, and in the bodies of premature infants fed cow colostrum at one Danish and two Chinese neonatal intensive care units (NICUs). Motivated by a scientific interest in gut microbiota and a translational ambition to improve clinical care, the establishment of NEOMUNE was intended to benefit Denmark by producing life, science, and capital concurrently. Now, NEOCOL will provide a platform for achieving this goal by applying NEOMUNE research results in ten NICUs in China.

As the day progresses, my attention drifts away from the PowerPoint presentations to the big black-and-white photographs from the middle of the twentieth century that decorate the walls along which the participants from China sit. One photo shows three white, male veterinarians (dressed in white coats and rubber boots) in a farm environment; another shows a cow undergoing some kind of medical procedure, with a group of veterinarians posing next to it; and a third shows a vet in a barn holding a newborn calf in his arms. The old building next door, constructed at the beginning of the twentieth century, is in the background of one of the photos. From previous meetings in this room, I know these old photos well. I have always read them as an expression of the Danish agribiopolitics that enabled the country's human population to thrive by governing populations of cows and pigs and fodder crops—resulting in the refinement of Danish butter, milk, bacon, pork loins, and other livestock products. In particular, the photos demonstrate the agricultural roots of the pig studies and my own and many of the researchers' connection to the agricultural field. Yet today, the discussion among the neonatologists about how to design clinical studies in high-tech medical settings in China does not include references to the historical background of pig studies and pork production. Although I know the connections to the preterm pig model, I cannot help thinking that the international neonatologists' talk of research design is a world apart from the Danish national ambition of optimizing the biology of production animals, as depicted in the photos. The photos portray a recent history, yet the latest research developments in the field make this history appear to be at an immense distance.

In this final chapter, I take my moment of reflection in the scientific seminar with international neonatologists in the historical Danish agricultural institution as the empirical starting point for tracing the path of cow colostrum across the border, as it leaves Denmark to produce infant health in Chinese NICUs. This path out of Denmark brings the border zones of species and life together with the geopolitical borders in my attempt to investigate questions about belonging. Historically, closing the physical borders of a nation-state has been an act of protection from enemies—be they unwelcome microbes from infected strangers, hostile soldiers wanting to conquer land, or pirates seeking to seize valuables. Simultaneously, open borders have been essential for exchanging commodities and generating value for society. In short, borders enable selection. They allow the entry of some things and some people and prevent the entry of others. They constitute not only zones of separation, but also zones of connection (Stasch 2009, 48). Here, I begin from the assumption that although physical barriers like seas, deserts, and mountains exist, these barriers are not in and of themselves natural borders. Rather, borders emerge through enactment (Van Reekum and Schinkel 2017, 27). As Laia Soto Bermant writes, "borders . . . ought to be understood as socio-spatial assemblages that produce the spaces they demarcate" (2017, 131).[1] The enactment of a border or a threshold illuminates how power works by including and excluding and how value is assessed in these dynamics. Today, when nonhuman things and animals move across national borders, such movements are referred to as importing and exporting—terms that represent such animals and things as objects of value generation. They can be owned and traded, and their movements into storage or the hands of new owners involve an act of value assessment and potential value generation. In contrast, migration refers to individuals who transport themselves to new destinations, and thus it entails a notion of autonomy that animals and things usually are not seen to possess. Nevertheless, as immigration politics illustrate, and as I discuss below, political efforts to close the national gates to migrating animals and humans reflect how the value and belonging of various animal and human lives is expressed in the enactment of borders.

In what follows, I rely on Kregg Hetherington's concept of agribiopolitics (2020) and Stefan Helmreich's concept of symbiopolitics (2009) to investigate under the same lens the movement of humans and nonhumans not usually put together: pork carcasses, cow colostrum, Argentinean soybeans, wild boars, and human migrants and refugees. I take an interest in how politics and public discussions about the crossings of these life-forms generate ideas about the welfare state as a metabolism that is positioned in an open interface of exchange with the rest of the world and that continuously filters material by admitting livestock products, humans, and animals seen as valuable, while keeping out those seen as a drain. Such images do not exist independently from social life. They have direct implications for how boundaries are enacted, how crossing is governed, and what is taken to be "society" and "environment." In the Danish setting, the national territory of Denmark is seen as equivalent to the welfare state. By focusing on policies that determine who and what may cross Danish national borders and enter the country, I pursue further the notion of the welfare state's sustainability introduced in chapter 3 and argue that the metabolic imaginary captures efforts to preserve the welfare state by securing, for example, high levels of health care, education, and social benefits for everyone, thus achieving a high level of equality among the state's human members. The metabolic imaginary is closely related to the Danish conceptualization of the work of citizens and the businesses run in Denmark as the sustenance of the welfare state: tax income and the activities of citizens are to be converted into welfare services (such as schools, hospitals, and other types of infrastructure) and create prosperous and fulfilling lives for citizens. In this imaginary, the societal organism is constantly constituted from the matter that flows through it. Within Denmark's borders, this view of mutual state-citizen relationships promotes a moral equivalence between participating in the labor market and welfare state institutions, on the one hand, and living a good life, on the other hand. By exploring policies and public discussions, I demonstrate that the goal of a fair conversion of resources into societal sustainability also involves selective permeability at the geopolitical borders. In connection to certain border crossings (research collaborations and the exporting and importing of agricultural products), policies and public discussions highlight porosity and interchange between environment and organism. And in connection to other border crossings (migrating wild boars and human migrants and refugees), policies and public discussions depict the Danish welfare state as a container that remains sustainable only by policing what can be taken in.

In this chapter, I draw on a number of written sources, particularly policies, reports, and newspaper articles. My reliance on these discursive sources means that I cannot show the lived experiences and the complexity of daily interactions at the geographical border that would be comparable to what I have been able to trace in the Newborn Pig Facility and the human NICU. What I wish to do by engaging policies and discourses across a variety of domains is to critically consider the wider social practices and discussions in Denmark from which the Newborn Pig Facility and the human NICU are inseparable. While political regulation and public discussions are certainly different from daily face-to-face interactions, I suggest that both policies and daily interactions may be conceptualized as practices of substitution. To recapitulate, in practices of substitution sociomaterial acts of replacement interweave moral and affective acts of stepping into the position of precarious beings. Where the previous chapters have described instances of substitution in the Newborn Pig Facility and the human NICU, in this chapter, I broaden the field and investigate how practices of substitution are systematized in politics and policies regulating movements across the geopolitical borders. I show that these politics and policies involve both assessing the extent to which the precarious life at the geopolitical border has the potential to substitute for original Danes (the sociomaterial component of substitution) and imagining and stepping into the situation of the precarious life in question (the moral and affective component of substitution). In turning attention to the policies and politics of geopolitical border crossings, I reveal how substitution practices materialize through an imaginary of the metabolic state and delineate the welfare state collectivity.

This book's investigation of liminality, substitution, and border crossings in relation to both pig and human neonates has continually brought refugees and migrants into view.[2] In this final chapter, I turn to refugees and migrants at the geopolitical borders to illuminate the symbiopolitical regulation of various liminal lives in the Danish welfare state. My argument is that the logics involved in substitution practices at the unsettled species borders in the Newborn Pig Facility and for human infants at the border between life and death in the NICU bear some similarities to the political regulation of refugees and migrants at Denmark's geographical borders. Just as substitution practices in the laboratory seek to turn research piglets into sustainable building blocks for society, immigration and integration policies involve practices of substitution that express the long-term aim of turning immigrants into sustenance for the welfare state metabolism. Moreover, the liminal lives of pigs and immigrants also intersect: immigrants who enter into a relationship with pigs by working on pig farms or eating pork enrich their potential for being metabolized and coming to belong.

First, I investigate activities, public discussions, and politics related to border crossings that have connections to Danish pork production. In this investigation I dig into the "historical lineage" (Cooper and Waldby 2014, 20) of the research piglets and the cow colostrum fed to them, as epitomized in the old photos in the seminar room. Second, I investigate how the Danish geopolitical border is imagined and enacted, at times as a porous membrane and at times as a fixed boundary. For instance, when animal products such as cow colostrum and Danish pork leave for China and when Eastern Europeans enter the country to take up work in the Danish pork production process, the geopolitical borders are made flexible or open. When migrating wild boars from Germany and human migrants and refugees from the global south move toward Denmark, the geopolitical borders are made inflexible or closed. Societal sustainability is seen as facilitated by porous borders in some cases, and by firm, protective borders in other cases. The political responses in different contexts reflect that in Denmark, belonging is closely connected with one's potential to enter the welfare state metabolism.

COW COLOSTRUM FOR CHINA

As a small country with an open economy, Denmark is highly dependent on foreign trade, and in the Danish imagination China has come to be seen as a particularly promising place to produce value. This opportunity is closely related to China's vastness and rapid economic growth. In the NEOMUNE and NEOCOL projects, setting up studies in China and introducing cow colostrum in Chinese NICUs are promising research activities because these institutions serve so many infants. Similarly, for Danish pork production firms, China is promising because it has so many people who eat pork.[3] Exporting Danish pork to China includes not only ordinary cuts of meat. Danish pigs' feet, ears, and intestines—in Denmark categorized as slaughterhouse waste—are delicacies in Chinese cuisine and are continuously shipped off to China. Moreover, in 2013, at the time the NEOMUNE platform received funding from Innovation Fund Denmark, the country's largest meat processing company, Danish Crown (known for its Tulip Sausages), became the first company in the world to obtain permission from the Chinese authorities to export processed pork to China. When permission for such exports was signed by the Danish minister of food and agriculture in 2013, it made eye-catching headlines in the national Danish media such as "Tulip Sausages Turn Over the Great Wall of China"[4] and "In China They Eat . . . Danish Sausages."[5] As the word "crown" refers to both the monarchy and the currency of Denmark, the name Danish Crown semantically connects pigs to Denmark's monarchy, king, and wealth—besides suggesting the premium quality of Danish pork. In a 2018 article about the growing market for Danish pork in China, the sales director at the Danish Agriculture and Food Council said, "China is a huge country of 1.4 billion people. If every Chinese person increases his/her daily intake of Danish pork with just four grams, this will double the Danish export of pork."[6] In September 2019, Danish Crown opened its first factory in China, which is expected to increase the consumption of Danish pork among the Chinese. All meat processed at the factory comes from Denmark, and the Danish minister of food and agriculture attended the opening ceremony. The minister's presence indicated that the Chinese market is not only a lucrative one for Danish pork producers, but also an important one for the Danish welfare state. Trade agreements are seen as creating pathways for Danish pork to move into China and transform into welfare for Danes.

Since 2018, the export of Danish pork to China has been bolstered by the unexpected actor of double-stranded DNA virus in the Asfarviridae family. This virus spread among domestic pigs in China and caused a major outbreak of African swine fever, resulting in the deaths of millions of Chinese pigs in 2018 and 2019 (Perrin and Bowen 2020) and a boom in the export of Danish Crown pork to China. Danish newspapers described Danish pork production as "hitting the jackpot" and the outbreak as a "game changer."[7] The combination of the double-stranded DNA virus and trade politics widened the gates for frozen meat from Europe and the United States to enter Asia and connected Danish pigs, pork production companies, and citizens to Chinese dinner tables and stomachs. The Danish media depicted Denmark as a community highly dependent on having porous boundaries between it and the surrounding world and included statements from political actors. The trade agreements treated a dynamic interaction between Denmark and the environment as crucial to converting Danish pigs into income for the Danish agricultural sector and welfare state.

Although in the NEOCOL seminar, I initially felt a distance between veterinarians working with Danish livestock in the barns and international neonatologists discussing the treatment of premature infants in the high-tech NICU environment, the coming together of these actors should not have surprised me. From the beginning of the industrialization of Danish agriculture, the goal was not only to feed the nation, but to do so by feeding the world. In the 2010s, the NEOMUNE and NEOCOL research platforms sought to contribute to achieving that goal by moving Danish cow colostrum from Biofiber, the Danish company, to Chinese NICUs. When this process began in December 2013, I entered a conference site outside Copenhagen and moved into the meeting room where a two-day NEOMUNE seminar was taking place. The faces of professors, postdoctoral and graduate students, animal technicians, clinicians, and industry partners shone with the enthusiasm and optimism that characterized the beginning of a new project.

One year earlier, we had received the good news that the funding application for establishing NEOMUNE had been approved. By the time of the seminar, most people had embarked on their projects, others had just been hired, and everyone was eager to network and engage with each other. The sixty people gathered for this event came from academic departments across the natural, medical, and social sciences; neonatology clinics in Denmark, Sweden, and the Netherlands; and the dairy industry. In his opening speech Professor Per the director of the Newborn Pig Facility and the NEOMUNE platform, said: "We will connect the gut and the brain and study how the gut affects the brain. We will conduct studies on mice, pigs, and infants. We will involve hospitals in

Copenhagen, Amsterdam, and Shenzhen in China. We do not only want to build knowledge, we also want to put it to use and achieve fewer infections, good digestion, and better cognition in premature infants." Professor Per's emphasis on connecting the gut and the brain by conducting studies across species, continents, lab and clinic, and basic and applied sciences came to be repeated in NEOMUNE meetings over the following years, and it was always invigorating.

In Professor Per's vision, knowledge about how the gut transforms carbohydrates, lipids, proteins, and amino acids and builds up cells in the brain is dependent on movements within a global field. He drew a picture of a world in which people and things can move freely and enter into relationships with one another. The translation of cow colostrum across farm, laboratory, and clinic was to be realized by fostering research collaborations across continents and introducing cow colostrum to populations of preterm infants in Chinese NICUs. His emphasis on the use and application of knowledge and the many actors he conjured up resonated with the goals of NEOMUNE's funder, Innovation Fund Denmark, which is concerned with creating value for Denmark in the form of "knowledge," "growth," or "jobs" (Innovation Fund Denmark, n.d.). The porosity of the borders of species, disciplines, institutions, and countries in Professor Per's talk can be interpreted as contributing to this aim of building Denmark up and securing its economic sustainability.

In the following years, NEOMUNE research facilitated collaborations across fields and paved the way for the NEOCOL project—which, like NEOMUNE, received prestigious and generous funding from Innovation Fund Denmark with the goal of creating value for Denmark. The aim of NEOCOL was to further realize the translational ambition through collaborations with ten NICUs in China, some of them three times the size of normal Danish NICUs. With this collaboration, the clinical pilot studies described in chapter 1 became a touchstone for clinical studies in which a minimum of 350 Chinese infants would be fed cow colostrum either as a supplement to mother's milk or as a replacement for formula.[8] To the Danish research team, the Chinese NICUs were valuable in several respects. First, they constituted a gateway to a very large population of neonates, and thus to a site where valuable NEOCOL data could be produced. Second, in Chinese NICUs, most preterm infants are fed formula—not their mother's milk or human donor milk, as is the case in Europe. This means that the collaboration with Chinese NICUs gave the researchers access to a population of infants in which it was possible to study and document the effects of cow colostrum compared to formula. Third, the clinical studies may establish a market for cow colostrum for infants that could be lucrative for Danish agribusinesses like Biofiber, which had extended its product range to include nutrition products for humans and spotted a market for these in China. Fourth, the collaboration made it possible for NEOCOL research to have a measurable impact on the health of Chinese infants, as the team expected the studies to show that cow colostrum is better at preventing NEC than formula.[9]

The Danish team was very aware of the ethical issues involved in this research. During the discussion among the international group of neonatologists in Copenhagen at the NEOCOL launch, one of the European neonatologists raised the concern that NEOCOL studies were not only taking advantage of the absence of mother's milk (including mother's colostrum) in Chinese NICUs but also maintaining this situation. She said, "Every mother will have colostrum. Full stop." An Australian colleague followed up: "It is ethically important to let the [Chinese] mothers know that their milk is better than any intervention." Swenyu, who was responsible for coordinating the studies, replied that the team always recommends mother's milk when talking to their Chinese collaborators, and that this has had positive effects. Through their years of collaboration with Chinese NICUs, breast-feeding has increased.

If we conceptualize the inclusion of Chinese infants in the NEOMUNE and NEOCOL research platforms as acts of substitution in which each infant (due to its common neonate biology) stands in for every other infant in the study, we also see that in this setting, substitution involves an affective dimension of asking what is best for the child and taking a moral stance. Whereas issues of outsourcing risk to poorer countries have been explored (Petryna 2009; Cooper and Waldby 2014), NEOMUNE and NEOCOL researchers did not merely intend to displace risk onto Chinese infants. The conversation in the seminar reveals that, on one hand, the Danish team capitalizes on the absence of mother's milk in Chinese NICUs. On the other hand, the team insists that mother's milk is best, and this advice works against the possibility of conducting long-term research that documents the effects of cow colostrum compared with formula in infants. Among Danish scientists and funders, the promise of the Chinese market pushes cow colostrum across the border along with advice that cow colostrum is not as good as the mother's own colostrum. We might see these moves as similar to the simultaneous acts of care and of use in the Newborn Pig Facility that I discussed in chapter 2.

In November 2017, ten months after the launch of the NEOCOL research platform in Copenhagen, I traveled to hospital sites in Shenzhen, China, where Danish cow colostrum would soon be given to Chinese neonates. On this trip to Shenzhen, the European NEOCOL group included Professor Per, three European neonatologists, two European scientists based in Denmark, one Chinese neonatologist who was doing his graduate studies in Denmark, one Chinese nutritional scientist who was doing his postdoctoral studies in Denmark, the director of Biofiber, the purchase manager of Biofiber, and me. The trip was one of Professor Per's many visits to China during the NEOMUNE research and demonstrates his dedication to collaborative relations. This dedication had involved inviting

Chinese neonatologists and scientists to Denmark and enrolling Chinese PhD students at the University of Copenhagen, where they were trained in running studies in the Newborn Pig Facility, gained access to data collected by the Danish team, wrote papers on these data, and were supervised by Professor Per and his senior staff. These migrating researchers were welcomed by Danish immigration policies—in contrast to other groups of human migrants. I next provide a short description of this trip from a Danish perspective.

On our second day we were to visit a women and children's hospital twenty kilometers from our hotel. From the taxi window, Shenzhen appeared as an endless array of gray skyscrapers, cars, and smog, and the traffic on the freeway was so slow that we would have moved faster on foot. Zhang, the Chinese neonatologist in our group who was now graduate student in Denmark, told me that less than twenty years before, Shenzhen had been a small fishing village in the Pearl River delta just north of Hong Kong. The status of Shenzhen as a "separate city"—meaning that it has more liberal legislation than mainland China does—had attracted foreign investments and businesses, especially technology firms. With a million new residents every year, the city had outgrown Hong Kong and had a population of thirteen million, according to official statistics. The majority of the population was under thirty, and thus many people were of childbearing age.

Arriving at the hospital, I looked at the huge buildings, each of which had 8–10 floors. Knowing that all this space accommodated only mothers and children and that this was just one of ten hospitals to be included in the NEOCOL studies, I began to realize just how large the study populations available in Shenzhen would be. As we moved inside and were shown around the NICUs, the Europeans could not help noticing and commenting on the contrasts to Danish NICUs. Compared to the typical Danish NICU, which had rooms for two infants and their parents, the average Chinese NICU was a huge area divided into sections, each of which accommodated more than twenty incubators that stood next to each other in long rows. One of my colleagues pointed out that there were no parent beds or parents present in the wards. As we continued through the NICU, another member of our group wondered aloud why there were no extremely premature infants, which are so common in Danish NICUs. Later in the day, Zhang explained to me that in China there is no obligation to save infants before twenty-eight weeks gestation. He explained that although parents can ask doctors to save an infant born at an earlier point, most parents are reluctant to raise a child with disabilities, due to insufficient health care in China and pressures on children to care for their parents in old age and do well in the competitive Chinese educational system. To me, the absence of tiny infants was evidence of "China's restrictive reproductive complex" (Wahlberg 2018, 8) and the country's intergenerational dependencies (Fong 2004) and "descending familism" (Yan 2016) that has created moral incentives and economic motives to invest as many resources as possible in the youngest generation. In short, reproductive policies and family structures shaped reproductive behaviors in different ways than in Denmark.

In meetings with staff members, the European group gave presentations of their research, and Gunner Jacobsen, the director of Biofiber, introduced the Chinese collaborators to the process of turning colostrum from Danish cows into a colostrum product for medical use in preterm babies. He showed photos of Danish cows in the fields and his company's high-tech production equipment used in pasteurization. All Danish and Chinese collaborators expressed great optimism about and engagement in the clinical studies, yet the meetings also uncovered the many cultural, practical, and epistemic challenges involved in setting up the clinical studies in China. Feeding regimes were repeatedly discussed. In Denmark, NICU infants are put on a fast feeding track, as growth is seen as a surrogate for functional health. In China, however, NICU infants are put on a slow feeding track to protect their guts. In Denmark, all preterm infants have access to mother's milk or human donor milk. But human donor milk is available in only two NICUs in Shenzhen, and many preterm infants are fed only formula designed for neonates.

In the context of these culturally conditioned organizational differences between the two settings, practical routines for clinical studies needed to be worked out. "Do you need containers for [the samples of the infants'] blood and feces? What about whisks to mix the cow colostrum fortifier and the milk? What about freezing space for blood samples and fecal samples?" the Danish neonatologists asked. "After every meal, we need to fill in this registration sheet and score the feces. How is this different from the registration you already do?" Along with all the practical issues, biological differences were mentioned. "Are Chinese and European children different genetically?" Professor Per asked. He suggested that maybe formula should be designed differently to suit different genetic profiles. The conversations clarified that the metabolic processes in an infant's body and the creation of data about these processes were inseparable from the politics of whose lives to save and include in society, clinical routines and feeding regimes, documentation procedures, the time available to staff members for registering food intake and taking samples, the time available to them for whipping colostrum, the availability of mother's milk and human donor milk, and the genetics of the children. Building a common kind of infant biology took much work and protracted negotiations.

If not for the ambition of participants in NEOMUNE and NEOCOL to create knowledge about this common kind of infant biology and move cow colostrum to NICUs across the world, these practical differences would not matter. Yet the project was based on the premise that scientifically it makes sense to compare gut microbiota and gut maturation of preterm infants around the world. This well-known idea of a specific, generic neonate biology embodies the idea that in principle infant bodies may stand in for each other—just as in the experimental practices pig bodies stand in for each other and for the infants who cannot be experimented on. Danish infants may substitute for Chinese infants and vice versa. As we saw in chapters 1 and 2, in the Newborn Pig Facility, the notion of generic infant biology resulted in discussions of the role of species in the studies. In meetings with the Chinese neonatologists and scientists, the same notion of generic infant biology resulted in discussions of the significance of local clinical routines and local biologies (Lock 2001) for the generated data. In witnessing the huge differences between clinical routines and treatment regimes in Denmark and China, the European neonatologists became increasingly skeptical about including Chinese NICUs in the same cohort as the Danish NICUs.[10] Although the NEOCOL project was based on the idea that cow colostrum provided feasible nutrition for preterm infants around the world and was preferable to formula-based products, at the end of the day, new boundaries between the data produced at the Danish and Chinese sites were erected to create homogeneous groups of infants within each study. In other words, boundaries were built as part of integrating the study sites in the NEOCOL research platform.

NEOMUNE and NEOCOL research was based on the porosity between gut and brain, and thus these studies acknowledge that metabolic pathways in infant bodies are entangled with exchanges between cows, pigs, and humans. This porosity resonates with Danish research and trade politics that imagine Denmark as a welfare state metabolism based on permeable boundaries with the world, through which agricultural products and students and researchers can move between Denmark and elsewhere. Yet the practices of setting up clinical studies across countries illuminate that flexible geopolitical borders for cow colostrum and Danish research teams do not necessarily mean that cow colostrum can be translated to the guts of Chinese children. Comparable sites are needed to build practices that can make Chinese and Danish infants mutually substitutable and convert the sustenance of cow colostrum into infant health, scientific prestige, and monetary income for Denmark. And comparable sites require whisks, fecal samples, containers, registration sheets, meetings, discussions about who can substitute for whom, and a change of local clinical routines in Chinese NICUs.

UNSETTLED BOUNDARIES

At the same time as cow colostrum and millions of tons of pork move across Danish borders to export markets, the large population of Danish pigs draws foreign products and bodies back across geopolitical borders. Porous boundaries to the world not only allow for the shipping of pork to foreign markets; they are also a precondition for raising twenty-six million pigs annually. In this section, I investigate how Danish production sows and the research piglets they produce are part of transnational relations that bring production pigs into intimate relations with Argentinean soybeans and human workers from Argentina and Eastern Europe. In analyzing these relations, I expose the agribiopolitical relations that regulate the flow of humans, pork, and plant crops across geopolitical borders.

Despite the facts that Denmark is one of the most intensively cultivated countries in the world and that fodder for pigs and other livestock dominates the crops grown in Danish fields,[11] Denmark still relies on importing animal fodder. The country imports 1.7 million tons of soybeans annually. Almost one-third of that amount (650,000 tons) consists of genetically modified soybeans from Argentina that are used to feed Danish pigs.[12] In Latin America, the production of soybeans for the global food market has dramatically changed the landscape and economy and created environmental concerns resulting from increased fires and the destruction of biodiversity in production (Changing Markets Foundation 2018). Additional issues are the health problems and deaths of workers because of the extended use of pesticides, as well as increasing poverty among farmworkers (Kregg Hetherington 2020; Lapegna 2016; Nepstad, Stickler, and Almeida 2006; Steward 2007), as big multinational firms dominate soybean production and concentrate profits in a relatively small number of hands (de Sousa and Vieira 2008, 238). Kregg Hetherington's ethnography of soybean production areas in Paraguay illuminates in unsettling ways the extent to which Latin American soybean production has resulted in the destruction of ecosystems and the loss of a way of life for the local populations—for whom soybeans have increasingly become "killer beans" (2013, 67)—while in other parts of the world this agribiopolitics is experienced in the form of an abundance of cheap meat (2020).

Soybeans for Danish pigs constitute a microscopic share of the Latin American soybean crop produced for the world market, and it is difficult to trace from which specific fields and corporations Danish pig farmers get their beans. Nevertheless, the importing of Argentinean soybeans for Danish pigs has resulted in critical reports from Danish investigative media.[13] In 2019, the import of soybeans resulted in an open consultation with the Danish minister of food and agriculture in which he had to answer critical questions from politicians in Parliament. The reports indicate that while the pig may look like a national health and welfare resource in Denmark, it draws upon and contributes to social inequalities and poor health and welfare among workers in Argentina, as well as playing a significant role in global climate crisis.

Although within the European Union (EU), Denmark takes a progressive stance and votes for sustainable food systems,[14] the use of imported soybeans in the Danish agricultural sector reflects how landscapes, soybean plants, and workers in Argentina become the "nonoptional company" (Haraway 2016, 115) of consumers of Danish pork.[15] In Denmark, the public became aware of how lean pork meat and revenues for the people occupying the natureculture (see the introduction) of Denmark were deeply entangled with high rates of cancer and congenital deformations among workers in Argentina due to the pesticide use that made it possible to expand cultivation of soybeans at the expense of other life-forms.[16] The transformation of Danish pork into welfare via soybeans and Argentinian workers, which came to the fore in the news reports and public discussions, made it difficult to determine where one body ends and another begins.[17] Porous passages between pigs in Denmark and landscapes and human lives in another part of the world were uncovered in unwelcome ways.

When it comes to human labor in the Danish pigpens, the work of sustaining the Danish pork industry also involves porous borders. Since the 2000s, the Danish agricultural sector has been increasingly populated with temporary workers from Eastern Europe. The Romanian workers whom we met on the farm in chapter 1 belong to a large group of intra-EU migrants who constitute one-third of all agricultural workers on Danish farms. This shift has happened in parallel with structural changes: formerly, large numbers of Danes owned and worked on their own small farms, but now a much smaller number of Danes own big agricultural production systems and employ an agricultural work force dominated by people from Poland, the Baltic countries, and Romania.[18] Many of the Eastern European farm workers in Denmark stay temporarily, returning to their home country after a couple of years.[19] When it comes to agriculture, Danish farmers have invited Eastern Europeans to their farms out of need. One report on the topic specifically states that Eastern European workers "substitute for Danish workers" (Jensen et al. 2007, 25).[20] Danish workers are no longer willing to take jobs in livestock production due to their low payment and inflexible work hours; the location of the work in remote areas; and the uncertain prospects for owning their own farms, as the intensification of production continues to concentrate the pig population on large farms.

In the Newborn Pig Facility and the human NICU, substitution practices unsettle borders of species and life and involve answering pressing questions about worthiness and belonging. When pig farms draw Eastern European workers across the geopolitical border onto Danish soil, they are welcomed as substitutes who stand in for the dwindling population of Danes willing to do farmwork. The Eastern European workers on Danish pig farms do not compete with Danes when it comes to performing the hard work in agriculture, and they literally optimize the pig resource of Denmark when they castrate screaming piglets without anesthesia, dock their tails,[21] remove dead piglets from the farrowing pens, or otherwise inhabit the space of compromise between animal welfare and profit making (Anneberg, Vaarst, and Bubandt 2013; Anneberg and Vaarst 2018; Hviid 2010). In the case of Eastern Europeans who substitute for Danish workers, to some extent the moral challenges of livestock production are being exported to EU migrant workers concurrently with the organizing of Danish farming into big livestock production systems. In contrast to other occupations, in farming there have been no public complaints about Eastern Europeans taking Danish jobs and no loud discussions of "welfare tourism"—a term that refers to the concern that EU citizens from less affluent countries move to take up work in EU countries with more generous welfare systems.[22]

Rather, in 2017, the director of the Danish Agriculture and Food Council declared that Eastern European workers "play a decisive role in the agricultural sector and that 'Production Denmark' cannot hang together without them."[23] The minister of occupation described Eastern European workers in Danish agriculture as "a condition for growth and welfare." One headline in a national newspaper read, "Our Welfare Cannot Do without Eastern European Workers."[24] These statements reflected the affective and moral component of substitution, as they demonstrated a moral stance on Eastern Europeans as valuable substitutes whom the Danish state welcomes and is ready to support in terms of providing welfare benefits. In political and public discussions, Eastern European farmworkers' contribution to Denmark is emphasized as a rationale for their belonging. Substitution provides a path into Denmark as long as the substitutes are seen as helping sustain the welfare state collectivity.

The agribiopolitical relations between Danish pigs, their fodder, and the workers involved in Argentina and Denmark present Denmark as a metabolism in which Danish pork chops or Danish cow colostrum for preterm infants are placed in relation to landscapes and bodies in different parts of the world. This metabolic image in which certain elements and organisms move in and out as part of creating a sustainable whole is part of both the positive story about Eastern Europeans getting work and saving Danish livestock production and the uncomfortable story about cheap pork chops at the dinner table being involved in environmental trouble and high rates of cancer and malformations among workers and their children in Argentina due to pesticide use. Both cases illustrate an imagination in which the permeability of the border is essential to producing Danish pork at the same time as the passages created through the border uncover how different precarious lives (e.g., production pigs in Denmark and farmworkers in Argentina) "interrelate in ways besides instrumental eating" (Solomon 2016, 227). When Denmark is imagined as a metabolism that sustains itself through exchanges, it becomes increasingly difficult to unambiguously categorize agricultural products as simply food for human and pig consumers. In other words, metabolic entanglements with other bodies contest any simple distinction between those lives that are worthy in and of themselves and those that are means to others.

SETTLED BOUNDARIES FOR PIGS

If porous boundaries at the national border connect the Danish welfare state to the world through agricultural production and trade agreements, other pig-related activities at geopolitical borders reflect a desire for strict gate policing that brings notions of belonging to the fore. To protect and maintain the high

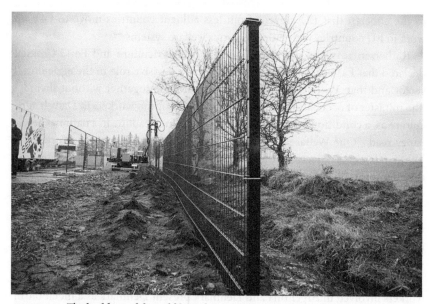

FIGURE 4.1. The building of the wild boar fence on the Danish-German border, 2019. Photo by Frank Cilius. (Credit: Frank Cilius.)

health status of Danish pigs and their extraordinary genes, highly restrictive rules regulate the importing of pigs from other countries. Concurrently with public articulations of pride about and praise for Danish sausages turning over the Great Wall of China, it is close to impossible for foreign pigs to enter Denmark and influence the Danish "breed wealth" (Franklin 2007, 47). Highly controlled breeding practices and the borders against foreign pigs illustrate the restrictive practices through which pigs are admitted into Denmark. Given that breeds connect bodies to place (Weiss 2016, 114), border policing for pigs adds value to the breed and brand of Danish pigs by filtering what does and does not belong in these animal forms.

However, wild boars occasionally cross the Danish-German land border on the Jutland peninsula. In 2018 as a response to the fear that African swine fever might reach Danish pig herds, the center-right government initiated the establishment of a fence that was seventy kilometers long and 1.5 meters high at the Danish-German land border (see figure 4.1).[25] The fear was not so much that wild boars would transmit the double-stranded Asfarviridae virus to Danish pigs and mate with them, thus threatening the biologically homogeneous population of domestic pigs. Rather, the main concern was that if wild boars on Danish territory carried the virus, Denmark would be classified as an affected zone—thus threatening the country's ability to export pork (Kristensen 2020, 10). At the same time as the virus assisted in opening the Chinese gates for Danish pork, Denmark built fences to protect itself from the virus.

The decision to build the fence was not unopposed. Critics pointed out that African swine fever does not exist in the countries neighboring Denmark, a fence would affect other wildlife in negative ways by disrupting species migration routes, a fence could not prevent wild boars from entering the country by water routes, and the risk of African swine fever's reaching Denmark comes from trucks transporting pigs across the border to slaughterhouses in Germany. Nevertheless, the Danish government did not want to take any risk at all. When the decision to build the fence was made, the minister of food from the center-right party argued, "If African swine fever reaches Denmark, an export worth 11 billion DKK [Danish crowns] will stop immediately."[26] The nationalist right-wing party, the Danish People's Party,[27] suggested adding a few meters to the fence's height to keep out illegal migration. However, German television and newspapers ridiculed the fence and compared it to President Donald Trump's fence along the U.S.-Mexican border.[28]

The anthropologist Sarah Ives writes that "the ecologically undesirable can easily merge into the demographically undesirable when people's claims to belonging are rooted in the soil" (2017, 109). The case of the pig fence exposes the contested politics of policing the ecologically, demographically, and commercially undesirable. In his analysis of social imaginations of society, Willem Schinkel notes that "underneath the usually unquestioned acceptance of 'society' as a kind of container of social life lies a continuous work of boundary maintenance and of sorting out of belonging" (2017, 5). In the fall of 2019, sorting out belonging did not only concern humans. Within the space of ten days, ten drowned wild boars were washed ashore Ærø, a small Danish island about twenty-five kilometers from the German coast. Experts did not see the drowning as a consequence of the fence,[29] and the Danish Veterinary and Food Administration decided to immediately remove and destroy the dead boars without testing them for African swine fever or other diseases. In the many newspaper articles on the incident,[30] the Danish Society for Nature Conservation stated its criticism of the decision that ran counter to the normal procedure and made it impossible to detect the cause of death and possible genetic connections between the ten animals. The Danish Veterinary and Food Administration explained that the reason not to test the animals was out of consideration for the Danish exporting of pork. In case African swine fever was identified in the wild boars, Denmark would have to announce internationally that the country was infected. Export losses would be unavoidable, even though no domestic pig was infected. A representative from the administration said, "These wild boars cannot be Danish, and the fact that they have been lying there on the beach does not put Danish piggeries at risk."[31] The situation was discussed at a meeting among member states at the European Parliament in Brussels, which supported Denmark's decision not to test the cadavers. Closing pathways for African swine fever by unknowing the reason of death was part of keeping the passage for pork out of Denmark open.

The political decision to establish the wild boar fence suggests an image of Denmark as a territorial container of people and pigs that needs to be segregated from a dangerous environment containing unwanted organisms. Here, porosity threatens to allow contaminating elements into Danish society, and closed borders become essential to societal sustainability. Yet in a world of porosity, fences cannot keep dead wild boars from washing ashore. The categorization of the animals as "not Danish," due to the fact that Ærø and the nearby island of Fyn do not have populations of wild boars, became an act of boundary maintenance—that is, of setting a boundary between a societal body and its environment. The establishment of the fence and the categorization of the drowned boars as non-Danish singled out pig bodies born on Danish land as the ones that rightfully belong in the natureculture of Denmark and are in a position to be metabolized by the welfare state. In contrast to local pigs raised to be converted to welfare for the collectivity, migrating wild foreign boars were articulated as putting the carefully balanced societal sustainability at risk. The political decision to abstain from testing the corpses enacted Denmark as a metabolism that has porous interactions with its environment and achieved sustainability by selectively regulating crossings at geopolitical borders.

SETTLED BOUNDARIES FOR HUMANS

To fully understand the scope of the metabolic imaginary, I now turn to policies and public discussions concerning human migration into Denmark. Pig and human immigration may at first sight seem unrelated to the research piglets in the laboratory and the production pigs on the farms. Nevertheless, bringing in immigration policies enables me to show how persistent the notion of the welfare state metabolism is across domains, and how it is articulated through substitution practices. This metabolic thinking affects not only the lives and deaths of pigs and humans within Denmark, but also the lives and deaths of human migrants at European borders. We have already seen how Eastern Europeans working on Danish farms are articulated as replacing—substituting for—Danish workers and doing important work in the welfare state. In this section, I expand this analysis by investigating how (human and pig) neonates and (human) migrants are imagined to be metabolized in ways that are not only parallel but to some extent also intertwined with each other.

Although the practices in the Newborn Pig Facility and human NICU are only indirectly connected to migration, the metabolic thinking in terms of what constitutes life-giving and life-draining material is also at stake when Emma, Peter, and Christian step into the position of Huxley, the limp piglet, and discuss whether or not to euthanize it (see chapter 2). In this situation, the researchers are concerned about how best to turn Huxley into potential for research funded by tax-financed institutions. Likewise, when Dr. Hans and Dr. Tina talk about their "societal responsibility" (see chapter 3), they balance the expected prospect for the infant with fair use of public resources and the infant's potential contributions to society, thus standing in a reciprocal relationship to the state. The near human in the border zones of species and viability and the lives of migrants at internal geopolitical borders activate substitution practices that regulate entrance. By keeping attention on the big picture (see chapter 3) and assessing the value of what is taken in and can be converted to health, happy family lives, and societal sustainability, the involved actors show and represent the welfare state as a metabolism.

Public discussion of immigrants' contributions to the welfare state and the welfare state's responsibilities for immigrants was already present in the nascent Danish welfare state in the 1960s. At that time, the import of Eastern European and Turkish so-called guest workers by the young Danish welfare state sparked public discussion about the extent to which guest workers should have access to benefits such as free health care, Danish lessons, and pensions (Jønsson 2018). As their name indicates, guest workers were seen as a temporary substitution by acting as extension of the Danish workforce. Immigration policies treated Danes as originals who authentically belonged in the country in contrast to guest workers—who, as substitutes, did not have full membership. We may see a parallel to the way parents of a very premature fragile infant saw their child as a guest who might stay in their lives only temporarily (see chapter 1). Both guest workers and infant visitors were positioned as liminal lives at the margins of either family or societal belonging. And practices of substitution that helped determine the futures of these guests and visitors provoked questions about attachment. In the NICU, the acts of substituting for premature precarious infants with uncertain prospects unsettled the borders between life and death and between temporary and permanent belonging and made parents uncertain about how best to attach to the infants. Similarly, discussions in the 1970s about guest workers' access to benefits concerned the extent to which the state should substitute for them. In this case, the discussion unsettled the border between guests and citizens and prompted questions about whether guest workers should be seen only as a workforce or as human beings in need of protections from the Danish state.[32] In 1973, as a response to the oil crisis and an increase in unemployment rates, Denmark stopped issuing work permits to such workers, yet the question of how to treat guest workers who were already in the country remained unresolved. In 1976 and 1977, guest workers from Turkey and Yugoslavia gained the same social rights as Danish citizens (Danish Ministry of External Affairs 1978, 1979). The rationale was that foreigners who had contributed to the Danish economy and paid their taxes were eligible for the same social security as Danish citizens were—even when work was difficult to find in less favorable economic times (Jønsson 2018, 28). Achieving reciprocal relationships between guest workers and the state was seen as a proof of their belonging in Denmark.

In the 1980s, Denmark issued a law granting close family members of immigrants the right to immigrate to Denmark.[33] In the 1990s, following the rise of family reunifications and an increase in the number of migrants from non-Western countries such as Vietnam, Chile, Iran, Sri Lanka, Lebanon, former Yugoslavia, Somalia, and stateless Palestinians, the political and public climate shifted, and Denmark tightened its immigration policies.[34] In the same period, European public discourses on immigration viewed Muslim migrants from the global south as the other. In Denmark, it became common to distinguish among categories of Danes—reflected in the recent concepts of ethnic Danes and new Danes—and political discussions and initiatives centered on better integration, a concept that depicts a "part" to be included in a "whole" and portrays immigrants as existing at a distance from society (Schinkel 2017, 36–43). In particular, the Danish People's Party supported a generous welfare state built exclusively for Danes. The concept of Danishness, along with discussions of the financial sustainability of providing universal social benefits, dominated the public immigration debate (Petersen and Jønsson 2013, 173–177).

In 2000, Denmark introduced the attachment requirement in its family migration policy targeting non-Danish residents and their incoming spouses. According to this requirement, family reunification could be obtained if the couple's "combined attachment to Denmark was at least equal to [their] combined attachment to any other country."[35] The attachment requirement treated some people as original Danes who naturally belonged in the country (their attachment is not questioned) and others (non-national couples) as people who do not belong but who may work on their attachment and come close to the original Danes. The selection implied in the attachment requirement has parallels to the way attachment operates in the NICU, where precarious infants' weak attachment to their family and the welfare state may hold a "discrete authority" (Navne and Svendsen 2019) in life-and-death decision-making processes and contribute to either moving infants at the margins of life across the border of viability or into palliative care. Yet, where life-and-death decision making in the NICU does not emphasize proximity to the original, the attachment requirement in immigration law creates a continuum in which equivalence to the original can be more or less. This parallels the way the research piglets are being assessed on their biological potential to be as close as possible to infants in the clinic. The moment piglets have no potential to substitute for the infant and contribute to the experiment, negotiations begin about when, if ever, to expel them from the experiment. Despite the huge differences between the situations, I see continuities. In all three cases, the expectations about these life-forms' contributions—in the form of happy family lives, promising research, and active membership in the community—shape decisions about their belonging.

Moreover, in the cases of the piglet and the incoming spouse, there is a limit to how close they can come to the original. In the Newborn Pig Facility, the inclusion of the piglets in the experiments rests on their being continuously modeled to become near human (the status that Danish research monkeys lost). In Danish immigration law since the early 2000s, the residence of migrants in Denmark depends not on their ability to become "original" Danes, but on their willingness to demonstrate their proximity to the original by acting as its extension. Thus, migrants who gain asylum can stay in the country only temporarily, and limits on the extent to which they should receive welfare benefits have become increasingly tightened. These selection policies do not operate only once for an individual—granting or refusing the person residence. Rather, national attachment becomes a "processual ideal" (Bissenbakker 2019, 192), as the law makes it increasingly difficult to reach the permanent residence and "natural" belonging status of the originals (Rytter 2010).[36] In his analysis of Dutch immigration discourses, Schinkel calls this way of regulating societal membership a "moralisation of citizenship" (2017, 33). Citizenship is not simply a set of formal rights. It is first and foremost something that can be earned by demonstrating particular behavior (e.g., passing language exams, being financially independent, and having a certain level of education), thus documenting national attachment. For immigrants who meet the criteria for particular kinds of belonging, paths across the Danish border can open.

At a dinner in 2015 for 50–60 NEOMUNE researchers, I ended up at a table with three postdoctoral students of Asian origin. One of them was Nhut, who had come to Denmark five years earlier to study for his master's degree and PhD. From NEOMUNE seminars I knew him to be an expert on the large-scale study of proteins using high-throughput methods, referred to as proteomics and transcriptomics. Earlier in the day he had given a talk that had received a lot of praise and admiration from the senior scholars present. While I had always seen Nhut as firmly belonging in NEOMUNE, the dinner conversation that night provided a glimpse into his uncertain societal belonging—which was in sharp contrast to my own unquestioned ethnic rootedness in Denmark. Nhut and the other two Asian scholars discussed the challenges they faced in gaining permanent residence, the loss and guilt related to leaving parents and siblings behind in their home countries, and their possibilities for caring for their parents in their old age. Less than two years later, Nhut received a five-year assistant professorship based on funding from the largest Danish dairy company. When I congratulated him, he told me that the position had secured permanent residence for him (as he was able to continue his employment), which meant that his wife could stay in Denmark. Had his employment come to an end, she would have had to leave. Her university degree from their home country was not acknowledged by the Danish authorities, however, and she had difficulty finding a job and earning a residence permit. He also reminded me that the requirements for permanent residence changed regularly. Just a month earlier, the requirement had been 6 years of residence and 2.5 years of employment out of the past 3 years, but it had changed to 8 years of residence and 3.5 years of employment out of the past 4 years. Nhut's story not only demonstrates the moralization of citizenship, which continuously placed him formally at the margins of society despite his central work in NEOMUNE; it also demonstrates that only people who are seen as providing sustenance for society can be considered eligible for permanent residence. In Nhut's case, literally laying his hands on pigs and translating their intestinal cultures into protein interaction networks became a way to enter the country permanently.

Unlike Nhut, many immigrants who wish to cross into Denmark do not meet these difficult criteria for entry. Particularly in these cases, the image of Denmark as a welfare state metabolism lends power and urgency to policies regulating which refugees and migrants to allow across the Danish border. Following unrest in the Middle East and Africa during the summer and fall of 2015, a huge number of refugees and migrants arrived in Europe. On the news in September 2015, Danes saw a sight never before encountered: refugees and migrants who had crossed into Denmark from Germany and were walking along the motorways to reach their Swedish destination. Fleeing from Syria, Afghanistan, Eritrea, and Somalia, they had passed the Hungarian border on packed trains or on foot and pushed their way to Germany and Northern Europe. In the Danish press, the pictures of these people, including children, with suitcases and backpacks walking on the motorway became icons of a changed world. Although many refugees and migrants wanted to simply pass through Denmark to reunite with family members and friends in Sweden—which at the time had a welcoming attitude toward refugees, especially from Syria—the event intensified an ongoing debate about economic sustainability and societal cohesion in the context of migration.

In the public debate, refugees and migrants were described as fellow human beings in need of refuge and care, and newspapers reported on Danes who left work and drove to the border to pick up refugees and transport them to the Swedish border. This was an unlawful act of human trafficking that could be punished with fines or prison sentences. Yet the public debate also portrayed refugees and migrants in other ways, as their ability and worthiness to belong in Denmark was constantly discussed. Should they be seen as saviors of the future welfare state, which was threatened by a diminishing workforce? Or were they undesirable elements undermining societal sustainability? Similar to the clinicians' discussions in the life-and-death border zone in the NICU, public discussions about how to portray and treat incoming migrants and refugees tacked between consideration for the needs of the individual person and the cost or benefit for society. The notion of Denmark as a welfare state metabolism came to the fore in these public conversations when refugees and migrants were viewed primarily through an economic lens, in which the humanitarian plight that Europe faced was subordinated to public fears that the economic burden of refugees and migrants threatened the sustainability of the Danish welfare state. In 2015 and 2016, the Danish People's Party played a decisive role in introducing temporary border controls along the Danish-German land border—including in the area where the wild boar fence was to be established a few years later—and catalyzing initiatives and regulations aimed at dissuading refugees and migrants from coming to Denmark.[37]

Concurrently, the EU reached an agreement with Turkey that every person from Turkey who arrived illegally in Greece would be returned to Turkey. In exchange, the EU gave Turkey huge sums of money to prevent irregular migration from Turkey to the EU and improve facilities for refugees in Turkey. While the deal externalized EU borders and significantly reduced the number of refugees arriving in Europe, it had grave consequences for refugees in both Greece and Turkey. In Greece, reception centers turned into detention camps overnight, and thousands of people ended up living for years in overcrowded containers and experiencing great suffering and legal insecurity. In Turkey, millions of refugees already lived below the poverty line, and with new people continuously being transferred from Greece, possibilities for refugees' forward movement were impeded.[38] Simultaneously, the EU cooperated with the Liberian coast guard to intercept refugees' water crossings to Europe. This resulted in an increase of people choosing more dangerous routes and living in disastrous conditions and provoked new forms of "border work" (Møhl 2020, 73) carried out by both migrants and EU border guards.[39]

Nicholas De Genova's depiction of "European deathscapes" (2017, 1) in the Mediterranean reminds us that only a small number of migrants and refugees eventually succeed in entering European societies. During the past ten years, thousands of dead bodies have been washed ashore in Italy and Tunisia or been found in overcrowded and unventilated shipping containers, while other people have died in slave-like camps in Northern Africa as a result of the EU's outsourcing its border policing to non-EU countries. The metabolic thinking at stake in the border enforcement at the margins of Europe produces a lethal distinction between those who belong and those who do not. The latter are no longer named guest workers but are called aliens, foreigners, or illegal migrants.

Many Danes do not feel that Denmark is complicit in the deaths of these migrants and refugees. Deaths at Europe's outer borders do not play a central role in Danish political discourse. For example, public discussions of the displaced persons' camps in Syria focus on Denmark's obligation to take back the few Danish citizens who left the country as foreign fighters and now live in the camps, not on the thousands of people remaining in such desperate conditions. In homing in on the threat to Denmark posed by foreign fighters, the discussions center on national coherence and sustainability.[40] I see this silencing of death at Europe's outer borders as closely related to the metabolic thinking in national politics. When Denmark is imagined as a welfare state metabolism that is continuously reconstituted by what it takes in and exchanges, then the estimated quality and character of the matter it imports from its surroundings becomes

crucial to its continuation. Viewed through this metabolic lens—or frame as Butler has it—migrants and refugees at Europe's borders come to appear as replace-
able and nongrievable.

The position that refugees and migrants left at the border must be kept out to
preserve the continuation of the welfare state was powerfully expressed by the
Danish minister of immigration and integration as a response to the situation at
the Greek-Turkish border in March 2020. At that time, Turkey was putting pressure on Europe to meet Turkey's demands by opening the EU border to migrants
and refugees. Thousands of migrants and refugees had crossed into Greece. The
Danish minister announced that the Danish government was ready to use the
"asylum brake" and said, "This brake allows us to temporarily close the border in
a situation of crisis."[41] The asylum brake was invented in a 2016 policy document
on regulating migration that was accepted by the government in that year. The
first sentences of the document read: "The Government pursues a consistent and
realistic immigration policy. We must render assistance in the world around us,
but we must also take care of Denmark. We must preserve our social cohesion
and values. And we must avoid putting too great a pressure on the local municipalities [responsible for integration of refugees into Danish society]" (Danish
Government 2016). Later that year, Mette Frederiksen, the leader of the opposition Social Democratic Party, who in 2019 became prime minister, said: "I don't
think that we can make society work if not everybody, who lives here, is integrated. Therefore, we must have a limit to the number we let in."[42]

Since 2015, this vocabulary of "tak[ing] care of Denmark," "preserv[ing] . . .
social cohesion," "avoid[ing] . . . pressure," and establishing "a limit to the number we let in" has strongly informed political discussions across the political
spectrum. In these discussions, arguments were made in favor settled borders,
with references to societal sustainability. The political rationale behind stricter
immigration policies was that by minimizing the flow of migration into Denmark, the state would have more resources for securing good integration for
first-, second-, and third-generation immigrants living in the country. Within
Denmark, the strict immigration policies have spurred public discussion of the
country's violating international conventions—for example, by preventing Syrian refugees to apply for family reunification in the first three years after their
arrival in the country and refusing to grant citizenship to the majority of disabled
people who applied for it.[43]

The Danish politicians' statements about access (limiting the number of
people let into Denmark) and integration (making sure that those admitted
become employed and embrace Danish culture), as well as immigration policies,
expressed a continuation in the treatment of immigrants arriving in Denmark as
substitutes in the sense that they were near yet possibly lesser than original
Danes. Yet in contrast to the guest workers in the 1960s and the Eastern Europeans in the present crossing the border to substitute for Danish workers on pig

farms, those fleeing from conflict and economic hardship were met with the sus-
picion that they could not contribute to society. Their belonging in Denmark
hinged on their ability not only to stand in for Danes, but also to produce value
for the welfare state—an ability that many politicians publicly doubted. We may
see these discussions as negotiations about whether to conceptualize migrants
as valuable substitutes who contribute to the metabolic processes of a welfare
state based on relations of solidarity or as life-draining material that threatens the
state's metabolic processes. This way of articulating "hierarchies of membership"
(Block 2015, 1434) shows that "borders do not exist only in physical proximity to
a borderline. Border-related spaces . . . also penetrate the wider society beyond
the material borderline, influencing both public debates and social, political, legal
and economic systems" (Olwig et al. 2020, 4). The Danish politics of belonging
concerned not only who to let into the country, but also how to assess and intervene in immigrants' connection to Denmark and their way of contributing to
society.

For example, in 2018 Parliament passed a law that made it mandatory for
children over the age of one who lived in low-income enclaves to attend public
kindergarten twenty-five hours a week. To let the state institutions take care of
preschool children is considered the normal way of life in Denmark.[44] The new
law was aimed at raising the number of children in day care among immigrant
families in an effort to regulate life in what the government officially called "ghettos."[45] The law claimed that children from such neighborhoods were "at risk of
growing up in parallel societies that have only minimal connection to Danish
society and only limited knowledge of the traditions, norms, and values that we
emphasize in this country. [Such limited knowledge] is problematic for the
children and youngsters' further journey in life—from day care to school and
education, and to the labor market" (Law on Education to Prevent Parallel
Societies 2018, 1). The aim of the law was to ensure that immigrant children "get
a good start in life" by improving their language skills and knowledge of Danish
values, which would optimize their school performance and future participation
in the labor market (Law on Obligatory Education Offer for One-Year-Olds in
Vulnerable Housing Areas May 28, 2018, Introduction). [46] For parents, noncom-
pliance with mandatory kindergarten could result in the termination of welfare
benefits. In addition, the law increased prison sentences for kindergarten leaders
who failed to report to the public authorities if they suspected that a child was
not thriving (*mistrives*).

These interventions point not only to a particular urgency in Denmark regarding who enters society, but also to a fear that immigrants and their children will
threaten societal cohesion. The law presents a majority "we" who hold specific
"traditions, norms, and values" to be equivalent to a moral citizenship. In opposition to this "we" stand immigrants who may have formal citizenship but who,
through their ways of living and their absence from welfare state institutions and

the labor market, are outsiders who should loosen their ties to "parallel socie-ties" and become properly attached to the welfare state collectivity. The law stip-ulates and enacts the form of substitution—replacement practices and moral and affective practices—discussed throughout this book. First, the law positions the immigrant child as a proxy for the moral Dane. Second, the law substitutes for the parents' upbringing by stepping in as the benevolent caretaker that knows what is best for the child. Here, Danishness—in the form of speaking the lan-guage, knowing Danish values and traditions, and becoming a future contributor to society—becomes crucial. In this practice of substitution, the common rights of parents in the welfare state are overruled. From the standpoint of the law, par-ticipation in public institutions, especially educational ones, is seen not as anti-thetical to personal freedom, but as the road to gaining personal freedom and having a good life within a collectivity of law-abiding Danish citizens. And achiev-ing that freedom and good life is a goal that justifies the temporary suspension of parents' basic rights. It may be that immigrants have Danish residence politically and formally, yet as Nhut reminded me, border controls in the form of new requirements and procedures are increasingly introduced to ensure that only valuable individuals gain access to lifelong social support and participation in the lifelong reciprocal relationship between state and citizen.

In the Newborn Pig Facility, making use of pigs is closely linked to keeping them alive for the duration of the experiment and "running the machine" (see chapter 2) of research within a public research institution. In Danish reproduc-tive politics and in life-and-death decision making in the NICU, infants are placed in webs of kinship and society and come to have intrinsic worth partly through being part of and of use to their family and society—entities that are seen not as antithetical to the individual infant but ultimately as an extension of it and oriented toward its own living. In the field of immigration, the law that made it mandatory for certain immigrant children to attend public kindergarten significantly spells out these logics. Here, entering kindergarten, school, and the labor market includes citizens into the collectivity, mutually shaping both the individuals and the welfare state metabolism on which they depend. By seeing life outside public day care as part of a "parallel society," thus representing a threat to the welfare state collectivity, the law portrayed children from low-income enclaves as potential deadweight that may shape the welfare state metabolism in unforeseen ways—for instance, by tipping the balance between securing resources for the state and providing universal services for citizens. In other words, migrants who do not enter the metabolic processes by participating in welfare state institutions, embracing Danish values, and generating income for the public purse are thought to endanger the continuity and maintenance of the collectivity.

While the notion of society as a bounded organism or metabolism is old,[47] it has taken center stage in Denmark's responses to human migration. If we view immigration and integration policies as practices of substitution, this form of substitution unsettles borders between belonging and not belonging, even after one is let into Denmark. In the field of immigration, practices of substitution involve weighing the potential of refugees and migrants to enter the societal metabolism by contributing economically and assimilating culturally. For some refugees and migrants caught up in the metabolic imaginary, borders are closed and asylum is refused. For those who are allowed in, immigration and integration policies position them as liminal lives "to get a good start in life" and be absorbed and transformed by the metabolic processes.

The political rationale for allowing soybeans and Eastern European workers to cross national borders reflects how the welfare state is imagined as a metabolic organism that sustains itself through a permeable interface with traffic. Yet migration policies and political discussions of what it takes for refugees and migrants to become part of the welfare state express the dangers of such porosity. The symbiopolitical relations that determine which crops, animals, and humans are allowed in or are rejected illuminate the fact that flow and stoppage are not antithetical.[48] Instead, they draw on and reinforce the same societal imagination and political logic of selective permeability.

PORK POLITICS

In public discussions about social insiders and outsiders, pork has come to play a role. Although Danes are ambivalent about the precarious lives in pig production and the pollution of Danish waterways from the slurry discharged at pig farms, pork is a staple part of many Danes' diets. In Denmark, pork is cheap. Pigs are considered ordinary production animals that contribute to the fabric of life.[49] When I spoke to friends and relatives about my research, many often told me that they did not eat very much pork. However, when I had lunch or dinner with the same people in their homes, I often found some kind of pork on the table. Even when pork was not the main dish, it appeared as bacon in the minced beef dish or on top of a vegetable soup, and it was served in meatballs made of a combination of pork and veal; hot dogs for the kids; or as pork liver pâté, sausages, or ham in lunch boxes. At cookouts, Danes barbecue all kinds of meat (including pork) and almost always serve pork sausages as an extra food that everyone would like, especially children. At birthday celebrations, hosts serve hot dogs as a good-bye meal after a full day (and night) of festivities.

My point is not that the people who say that they do not eat a lot of pork are deliberately lying. Rather, pork is ubiquitous in Danish cooking, and at the same time it is unremarkable. Not only do Danish pigs live off Danish (and Latin American) soil, but pigs also constitute the soil of Denmark to such an extent that they are an unnoticed ingredient in daily cooking, family life, and public spaces. An illustration of pork as a basic food in a public space is the Danish hot dog stand, called *pølsevogn*. This hand-pulled sausage cart is found on public squares or street corners in most Danish towns and cities. The *pølsevogn* has existed since 1910 and continues to constitute a recognizable part of urban settings. It shows that the pork-based sausage is not only a basic food that is always available (the hot dog stand is often open until late in the evening) but is also something connected to everyday conversations and socialization. At the *pølsevogn* you take a break, eat the sausage, and chat with the *pølsemand* (the person selling the sausage) and engage in small exchanges with other customers.

In 2007, the Danish People's Party suggested that to protect Danish culture in the context of Muslim immigrants in the country, the food served in public institutions such as nurseries, kindergartens, and nursing homes should include traditional Danish meat pâtés and meatballs based on pork.[50] The discussion resumed five years later, and this time Prime Minister Helle Thorning-Schmidt, a Social Democrat, entered the debate and warned against "slowly letting Danish food traditions slip out of public institutions."[51] As part of this long-running debate—dubbed the "meatball war"—in 2016 one municipality voted to mandate the serving of pork in taxpayer-funded nursing homes, schools, and day care centers. This was to ensure that "Danish food culture remains part of public institutions," as one local politician said.[52] Kenneth Kristensen Berth, a member of Parliament from the Danish People's Party, made a similar link to Danish history and culture, arguing that "it [pork] is part of our history and traditional Danish cooking. It is unacceptable that meat balls are based on chicken" and suggesting that "We need a kind of pork rationing so that pork is served as a minimum once a week. We need legislation to secure a menu that takes consideration of Danes in both schools and day care."[53] These statements suggest a metonymic relationship between Danish culture, pigs, and Danish institutions through which human, pig, and state become an emotive moral whole.[54] The use of pork-based Curosurf and heparin in Danish health care (see the introduction) might express a similar connectedness between pig and human, yet the use of pork in these medications has not become public knowledge or been connected to the moral whole of the welfare state collectivity. This was different in the case of pork as a dietary product. Proponents of compulsory pork intake imbued a pork diet with values of authenticity and cultural heritage by linking it to the Danish pig soil. The public discussions about the menu in Danish public institutions point to what we also saw in the discussions of the boar fence—namely, an enactment of the welfare state collectivity as not simply a sociality of humans, but as a natureculture.

The "meatball war" was the subject of one editorial after another in Danish newspapers for more than ten years. An often-voiced criticism of the requirement to serve pork in public institutions was that decisions about what to serve were properly made by the local boards of, for instance, day care institutions, and that day care institutions in multicultural areas in Copenhagen had not experienced any controversies when they had decided to take pork off the menu. To explain her position, one nursery director said, "We have chosen to serve halal meat based on an ambition of inclusion. . . . In this institution, we have children from many different cultures, and it is important that what we eat is a shared experience. Children need to experience mutual connection. . . . We take care of many children and have a responsibility, [including] a responsibility for them to be part of a community."[55] Despite holding the opposite view of the people advocating for the mandatory serving of pork, the nursery director shared her opponents' concern about societal cohesion and belonging in the community. Yet to her, belonging was connected not to the consumption of pork in public institutions but to sharing and eating the same food (no matter what its origin) in public institutions.

The political suggestion to mandate serving pork treats the consumption of pork as a gateway into Danish welfare institutions in the sense that eating pork marks those who can pass and legitimately become part of the collectivity. What I find remarkable about the debate is that it goes uncontested that eating pork is a sign of belonging in Denmark. In the discursive space of the public debate, it would be absurd to say that eating pork signifies not being Danish. The debate is based on the assumption that eating pork is a default mode of being Danish, identifying both those whose belonging is unquestionable and those whose belonging may be questioned. In other words, having the right connection to the pig—by working on the front line of industrial pig farming, turning the pig into an object of science, or absorbing pork at the dinner table—provides a legitimate gateway to moral citizenship. If we see absorption as "the possibility for bodies, substances, and environments to mingle" (Solomon 2016, 5; see also chapter 1), then Danish pork politics suggests that taking in pork creates an absorptive interface of person, animal, and welfare state collectivity in which national belonging can be crafted. Consequently, at the same time as the dominant position of the pig in Denmark is that of a cheap, low-status production animal, its identity simply as food imbues it with the power to differentiate belonging. Danish pigs represent not only an economic resource. Some voices in the public debate also give pigs the role of determining who may rightfully use welfare state infrastructures and occupy welfare state institutions, be it the motorway or the kindergarten. For both people and pigs, bearing the marker of Danishness and manifesting a relationship to the Danish pig soil confirm belonging in the welfare state collectivity.

METABOLIZING LIFE

In 2014, a Danish newspaper article described exporting to China Danish knowledge about how to run nursing homes and nurseries and how to dispose of wastewater as "the new bacon."[56] Hinting at the significant role that bacon exports to Britain played for the Danish economy and welfare in the twentieth century, the "new bacon" epitomizes the pig as the product that becomes a crucial societal resource by crossing Danish borders. In the twenty-first century, the welfare infrastructures that were built with income from agribusiness have turned into a potential resource for generating wealth and welfare for Denmark.

The story about the "new bacon" raises questions about what can become a resource. As Elizabeth Ferry and Mandana Limbert argue, "Nothing is essentially and self-evidently a resource" (2008, 4). Rather, the concept of resource entails "ideas of the world as available for human use, and of that use as the basis of proper human society" (8). This chapter reveals that in the Danish case, what can become a resource is determined with an eye to producing a sustainable welfare state collectivity. The policies and public discussions I have scrutinized reflect an imagination of the welfare state as a metabolism in which policies are positioned as ways to sustain its existence—which is seen as ultimately in the service of providing good lives for residents. In this metabolic imaginary, the uptake of human and nonhuman resources and their conversion into welfare for citizens is "proper human society." This imaginary simultaneously delineates an external world, thus distinguishing Denmark from its surroundings. The human tragedies outside Denmark, which this societal imagination produces through selective practices of inclusion (of soybeans from Argentina) and exclusion (of humans at the EU peripheries), are not silenced in public discussions, yet they do not lead to a change of border practices. The powerful metabolic thinking in the Danish welfare state is pervasive and operates across domains in a way that naturalizes selective permeability. In Danish public discussions about what may enter or leave Denmark, the idea of economic sustainability to some extent is transformed into moral sustainability: the person who is in a position to be metabolized by contributing to the public purse and standing in a reciprocal relationship to the state and the tax-paying collectivity gains the marker of belonging. Moreover, since the pig is seen as a basic societal resource, in some situations it becomes a kind of arbitrator that unveils the boundary between what and who belongs and can cross into Denmark, and what and who does not belong and should stay outside. For people and products entering Denmark, an alliance with Danish pigs strengthens their metabolizing potential.

In the geopolitical border zones—where international clinical studies are initiated, agreements on trade are made, fences are built, and immigration policies are tightened—imaginations of the relationship between a societal organism and its environment are anything but stable. Here policies regulating who and what can cross the geopolitical borders constitute substitution practices that enact the welfare state as a metabolic process that has permeable interfaces with the outside world. Only through engaging in activities of exchange with its surroundings can it exist and maintain itself. When porosity is seen as extending the conversion of resources into national welfare, porous boundaries are embraced. When porous boundaries are seen as a threat to the sustainability of the societal metabolism, the notion of the welfare state as a container is embraced, and closed gates are seen as crucial to securing national welfare.

The symbiopolitics that comes to the fore in the controversies about the regulation of geographical borders for pigs and humans draws the contours of a welfare state in which the prospect of becoming a citizen is connected to entering reciprocal economic and cultural relationships with a welfare state collectivity across the life span. By articulating societal sustainability as a concern, human and animal immigration policies in some ways parallel life-and-death decision making in the Newborn Pig Facility and the human NICU. Moreover, by identifying what can be a resource for "proper human society," migration policies reflect past polices of eugenics and present policies on prenatal screening (see chapter 3). Whereas in the 1930s, unregulated reproduction among the unfit caused moral panic among the middle classes and led to dramatic measures of reproductive control, today unregulated immigration from the Middle East provokes comparable regimes of control. Migrants are now the ones who are seen as threatening societal cohesion. In the period between the 1930s and the 1960s, eugenic policies coexisted with, and formed the precondition for, policies that provided citizens with social benefits in case of illness and unemployment. Today, restricted access to the welfare state goes hand in hand with interventions that promise citizens equal opportunities. The metabolic thinking across domains reveals the notion of selective permeability at the heart of governing borders. Practices of filtering lives are perceived as part of maintaining universal welfare services for those who occupy reciprocal relationships with the Danish state. The ideal of maintaining an egalitarian society in which everyone is placed in a mutual relationship with each other and the state becomes a vehicle for practices of differentiation. In policies and public discussions, caring for some implies the exclusion of others, and for those who enter there is no strict distinction between constituting a means and constituting an end. Across the sites of the animal laboratory, human clinic, and integration policies, substitution practices erase a clear distinction between instrumental and intrinsic worth. The human who has metabolizing potential easily gains intrinsic worth. Being metabolized increases the chances of coming to belong. The symbiopolitical governance of relations among entangled beings is directly linked to the ambition of sustaining equal life opportunities and high levels of universal care for humans who have already been let into Denmark. The near human figure in the border zone is not marginal to the welfare state. Rather, observing this border figure takes us to the very center of the processes that define the species and life-forms that belong in Denmark.

EPILOGUE

In March 2020, as I write these lines, human-animal entanglements and practices of substitution are unfolding before my eyes in new and profound ways. A week ago, the World Health Organization formally declared the outbreak of COVID-19 a pandemic. It has spread across continents, causing illness, death, and economic crisis in a world reliant on extensive flows of people and goods across national borders. While the species in which the virus originated is still not known, there seems no doubt that it has the bat as a source and probably also an intermediate animal host, thus illustrating the porous borders between species. Now that the coronavirus has reached human bodies without any immunity, thousands of people hover between life and death, and national health care systems fear or already face a deficiency of test kits, intensive care beds, respirators, and qualified staff members. Porous species borders intersect with porous borders between life and death. Reports from China and Italy, which were the first places to experience overloaded health care systems, reveal the critical and ubiquitous presence of the question at the heart of this book: whose lives are worth saving?

To be in a position to accommodate treatment for as many COVID-19 patients as possible and avoid being forced to choose between them, on March 11 Denmark became one of the first countries in Europe to close down all schools, universities, and other public institutions. A few days later, the Danish prime minister declared the national borders closed for travelers who did not have a legitimate reason (such as working or living in Denmark, delivering goods to Denmark, or visiting very sick relatives there) to enter the country. The prime minister also asked all Danish citizens abroad to return to Denmark unless they had permanent residency in another country. While COVID-19 is new, the strategies to deal with it are old and echo the kind of border work we have seen throughout this book: an enactment of Denmark as a welfare state metabolism that selectively allows some elements in and keeps others out. At the German-Danish borders, selective permeability materialized when goods and Danish citizens could freely move into and out of Denmark, while people with no legitimate reason to enter were turned around. The political actions of closing the country down and closing its borders gained strong public support. Concurrently, Danish hospitals prepared for the expected inrush of infected patients in need of care, and politicians took action to support businesses suffering from the lockdown.

The jumping of a virus from animal to human and from human to human in a globalized world unmasks the interconnectedness of lives and the unboundedness of bodies. If kinship refers to "a mutuality of being" (Sahlins 2011, 2), the pandemic demonstrates that "all earthlings are kin in the deepest sense" (Haraway 2016, 103) and shows the virulent—and deadly—potential of interspecies kinship. At the same time, governmental responses of closing national borders and asking people to maintain social distancing reveal that essential to human survival is not only kinship "in the deepest sense," but also the erection of borders "in the deepest sense." As the Danish prime minister phrased it, "we need to stand together by keeping [our] distance" (*Nu skal vi stå sammen ved at holde afstand*) (Frederiksen 2020a). This directive implicates porosity and entanglement between earthlings as the ground on which we stand, while it commands us to erect borders between nations and bodies so that our species can remain alive. In this sense, COVID-19 crystallizes the dual processes of entanglement and boundary making that I have explored in this book and invites us to investigate the border zone anew as a crucial site for constituting and valuating life.

In Denmark, the political efforts to curb the invisible coronavirus demonstrate once again how the "me" and "we" are crafted simultaneously through substitution, as well as showing who is excluded. The Danish political responses to COVID-19 aims to increase the number of respirators to take over sick citizens' failing lungs, enabling health authorities to enforce treatment and quarantine in connection to the virus outbreak, and providing economic support to the many Danish citizens who have lost their businesses and incomes due to the lockdown. We may see these measures as what I have named the sociomaterial practices of substitution. Concurrently, the political responses raise questions about the moral responsibilities arising from connectedness and entanglements. In short, who is to be protected and kept alive? Who belongs in the collectivity? The ambivalent act of struggling with these questions constitutes what I have referred to as the affective and moral component of substitution. In Denmark, the closing of national borders for anyone without a legitimate reason to enter the country offers one kind of answer to these questions. The virus was depicted as literally life-draining material that threatened the welfare state's possibilities for substituting for citizens' lives, thus prompting the closing down of borders. However, the virus had already entered the country as an invisible passenger on traveling citizens and was already spreading among humans and animals. A week into the lockdown, it appeared that closing the borders was not supported by the Danish health authorities. As a purely political action without medical evidence to support it, the border closing strongly communicated that in this moment of crisis, the sustainability of the welfare state metabolism relied on a connectedness—a kin relationship—between the Danish state and its citizens within its national geographical borders.

On national television, the Danish prime minister encouraged the nation to show "community spirit" (*samfundssind*), as she put it (Frederiksen 2020b). Furthermore, with this concept, she activated the strong ethos of relations of solidarity and cooperation in a national welfare state collectivity. She also spoke clearly about the state "holding up" (*holde hånden under*) Danish employees and businesses, thus portraying the state as literally sustaining (substituting for) citizens' lives and suffering businesses. She presented the vision that from life's beginning to its end, the welfare state cares for its citizens. In this vision, the state and the citizen belong in the same household (or metabolic system), in which the continuous respiration of citizens constitutes the continuous life and sustainability of the welfare state. As COVID-19 puts the elderly population at particular risk, one might have expected a virus-caused elimination of old "less productive" lives to be welcomed in a country envisioned as a welfare state metabolism. This was not the case. Once again, policing the geopolitical borders was seen as crucial to sustain the welfare state and make it live up to the reciprocity of state-citizen relationships, in which those who have paid taxes through a lifetime can expect care through a lifetime.

On the day of the border closure, Danish media showed pictures of huge concrete blocks in front of ten of the thirteen Danish-German border gates in the same area as the wild boar fence, all deployed to keep the virus out and ensure the state's ability to substitute for citizens. The concrete blocks at the Danish borders clearly showed how practices of substitution actualize questions of belonging and enact exclusions. While the Nordic countries are often viewed as having achieved an ideal kind of equality, this book's documentation of the selective reproduction and migration policies accompanying this achievement are rarely talked about on a global stage. My attention to what it takes to turn neonates into biographical and biological lives illuminates how excluding lives has been part of building up one of the most egalitarian societies in the world. As I write, several nongovernmental organizations are warning that the border shutdowns all over Europe impede aid from reaching refugee camps at Europe's borders and that a COVID-19 outbreak in refugee camps may cause huge numbers of deaths. Every country's use of its attention to its own citizens' health as a justification for closing national borders profoundly demonstrates how "belonging ... always relies on exclusions" (Gammeltoft 2014, 235). The arms that "hold up," in the prime minister's words, do not substitute for every human and animal. The agribiopolitical and symbiopolitical relations I have excavated in this book reveal a national politics of belonging that organizes attachment to the welfare state collectivity in terms of reciprocal relationships. Concurrently, I have demonstrated that as populations of pig and human neonates are included in the welfare state collectivity, the symbiopolitical governance of relations draws moral divisions between them.

If substitution exposes the coexistence of entanglements and border work, what lessons can be learned about what it takes to become a certain form of life? I started this book with my friend airing her surprise at my interest in pigs. Her "just a pig" comment alerted me to what is involved in constituting life and its worth. While this question of life's worth is instantly recognizable in the context of humans, it is less common to move across species and raise the same question in connection to pigs. Yet moving between the sites of the Newborn Pig Facility and human NICU drew my attention to the social, temporal, and spatial arrangements it takes to become a certain form of life and gain particular kinds of worth. If initially I saw the concept of substitution as a way to grasp animal modeling, substitution turned out to be an aperture in excavating formations and cessations of species, life, care, and belonging. Substituting for liminal lives attunes us to the porosity both of the human as bodily constituted through exchanges with the world and of the human as normative category that accommodates some lives and excludes others in particular situations and historical circumstances. Moreover, practices of substitution spell out the simultaneous processes of associating human value with originality and constituting human value through replacement. We are brought back to Emmanuel Lévinas's point that substitution is integral to becoming "the I, the unique one" (1974, 117). It is through being substituted for that neonates come to appear as originals and biographical lives. It is through being substituted for that patients with COVID-19 may once again become able-bodied citizens.

This relationality of life and its value has been well documented. Ethnographers and philosophers have long noted that humans' vulnerability and dependence on others are not the exception but central features of life and death. Scholars who highlight this interdependence argue against the ontological notion of human autonomy and show us instead how social, moral, and technological relationships make us stay in life. In a similar way, the research I have presented in this book highlights how preterm infants are highly dependent on research piglets, technologies and skilled expertise, parents who are willing to care for them, and a health care system that is ready to deal with them. As depicted in the reproduction of Patricia Piccinini's Undivided on the book's cover, the animal-like creature and the boy in the bed are connected through care and intimacy. Yet this book's explorations of research and clinical practices and welfare politics in the past and present should not lull us into seeing interdependence as always life-supportive and life-giving. As much as practices of substitution unsettle boundaries and highlight interconnectedness, they also involve drawing boundaries and selecting and sometimes discarding lives. Substitution practices give or deny the worth of liminal lives by incorporating them into species, life or death, and categories of belonging or not belonging. In these practices, difficult ethical questions across species illuminate that life's worth is a precarious achievement. Moreover, this book's movements across experimental, clinical, and political fields reveal that intrinsic and instrumental worth are not ontologically irreconcilable, although they are often seen as opposite in Western thinking. In practices of substitution in which professionals negotiated the entry of piglets and infants into society, the distinction between instrumental and intrinsic worth was often destabilized. When piglets gained potential to become means for scientific advancements, they also gained the potential to become grievable biographical lives. When infants were seen as means for good family life and a sustainable welfare state, they became ends in themselves that had intrinsic worth. When migrants were seen as sustenance for the welfare state metabolism, welfare state policies treated them as worthy of belonging. Reciprocal exchange relationships thus become pivotal to defining worth and suspend a clear distinction between instrumental and intrinsic worth. In the Danish case, intrinsic and instrumental worth do not simply coexist; instead, they condition each other.

In contrast to a strong trend in medical anthropology that focuses on disadvantaged people who are suffering and deprived of basic rights and care, this book has investigated the management of precarious lives in a highly privileged context. I have situated myself in the Danish majority population among professionals who are part of a thoroughly benevolent endeavor (saving human lives, taking good care of research animals, and creating good science) supported by taxes paid by people who live in one of the most egalitarian societies in the world. Nevertheless, stepping close to these processes illuminates the moral complexity that occurs when different liminal lives become interlaced. The substitution practices I have excavated in this book show that efforts to sustain and substitute for one liminal life (the vulnerable infant) cause suffering for another liminal life (the piglet). Likewise, political efforts to substitute for people at risk of COVID-19 become a justification for closing European borders, contributing to the peril of refugees and migrants attempting to enter the welfare state. Who and what is the vulnerable part—and who and what is original or substitute— cannot be taken for granted. Rather than operating with a fixed idea about whose lives are worth living and supporting, I have taken a different route. By moving across human and pig and across different kinds of humans (i.e., infants and migrants) I have uncovered how questions about the worth of lives emerge when professionals care for the future of both the individual (pig or human) and a greater collectivity. In particular, these practices unsettle commonsense understandings of equality by bringing to the fore notions of solidarity and sustainability in practices of exclusion.

The notion *Near Human* has helped me open the ethnographic field and draw attention to and inhabit the border zones where life and categories are in flux. As much as this notion has guided me in unravelling substitution practices, my documentation of the tangled lives of research piglets and preterm infants uproots the concepts of human and society as predetermined entities in the world and encourages us to focus on the boundary-making practices that bring human and society into being in the first place. Rather than seeing action as already grounded in human and society, we should direct our analytical attention to how these phenomena are configured and come to shape life and living. In particular, I see my multispecies and multisited approach as having the potential for uncovering how the human is configured and how society and its borders are continuously enacted. This methodology of juxtaposition pushes us toward the edge of our political comfort zones and opens a space for unraveling the ethical field of substitution. In my specific case, moving across different human and animal lives and across domains has rendered visible the social, spatial, and temporal arrangement of drawing liminal lives into dimensions of biography and personhood and manifesting the Danish welfare state at the edges of life. This method of moving across species and dissimilar spaces makes it possible to glimpse how human and society come into being and how human and animal create conditions of possibility for one another.

ACKNOWLEDGMENTS

Every book is a result of collaborations and an extended network of relations. Yet I feel that the relational and collaborative character of *Near Human* is particularly important. The idea of investigating the role of the Danish pigs in medical science was born in numerous conversations with Professor Lene Koch, who has been my mentor and collaborator for more than twenty years. In 2009, we embarked on a joint project on human-animal relations in medical science, which has laid the ground for *Near Human*. I am deeply indebted to Lene for being my closest discussion partner and reader. Every insight in this book bears the trace of our companionship.

Animals in laboratory spaces and infants in intensive care are not easily accessible to outsiders. In the animal facility, I am deeply indebted to Professor Per Torp Sangild, Professor Thomas Thymann, and Associate Professor Stine Brandt Bering for opening the door to their research practices, engaging with my anthropological methods and perspectives, and inviting me in as partner in the NEOMUNE project. Thank you to the whole NEOMUNE team for always welcoming me and trying to answer my odd questions. Heartfelt thanks to Mette Viberg Østergaard, who took me by the hand and introduced me to a world of piglet biology and laboratory practices in my early years of fieldwork. In the neonatal intensive care unit, Professor Gorm Greisen and Chief Surgeon Steen Hertel generously invited me into its busy clinical life and were always ready to engage with my questions and issues beyond a strictly medical perspective. I am truly grateful to all of you. I also thank Gunner Jacobsen, director of Biofiber-Damino, and his welcoming staff members, who helped me understand the many steps involved in converting cow colostrum to human nutrition.

The ethnography and analyses in the book have been developed in collaboration with the LifeWorth team: Professor Lene Koch; Mie Seest Dam and Iben Mundbjerg Gjødsbøl, former graduate students who are now assistant professors; Laura Emdal Navne, a former graduate student who is now a senior researcher; and Associate Professor Anja Bornø Jensen, who joined the project at a later stage than the others did. Our joint exploration of the ethical and existential questions related to taking care of precarious human and animal lives has constituted the magic of my working life and shown me the great excitement that comes with working as a team. By taking seriously the fact that interdependence is a condition of not only the precarious lives we investigated but also of academic life, we dared engage the awkward juxtapositions on which this book stands.

My research was made possible by grants from Independent Research Fund Denmark (Grant 09-065723 and Sapere Aude Grant 12-133657) and Innovation

Fund Denmark (through the NEOMUNE research platform), and a major part of the writing took place in connection with my grant from the Carlsberg Foundation (Semper Ardens Grant CF17-0016). Thanks to these resources, I had the opportunity to form the LifeWorth team and form relationships with scholars in the fields of medical anthropology and science and technology studies in Europe and the United States. This book is firmly situated in my close relationships with a large group of scholars who have engaged in conversations with me and read drafts of the book or the published articles on which it draws. They are Erica Borgstrom, Annamaria Carusi, Nancy Chen, Astrid Christoffersen-Deb, Simon Cohn, Jason De Léon, Tone Druglitrø, Marieke van Eijk, Susan Erikson, Carrie Friese, Tine Gammeltoft, Faye Ginsberg, Lone Grøn, Stefan Helmreich, Amy Hinterberger, Linda Hogle, Sharon Kaufman, Claas Kirchhelle, Rob Kirk, Teresa Kuan, Joanna Latimer, Francis Lee, Emily Martin, Andrew Mathews, Cheryl Mattingly, Lotte Meinert, Perle Møhl, Annemarie Mol, Lynn Morgan, Michael Montoya, Laura Emdal Navne, Nicole Nelson, Adriana Petryna, Vibeke Pihl, Jeannette Pols, Barbara Prainsack, Lillian Prueher, Rayna Rapp, Jenny Reardon, Tobias Rees, Andreas Roepstorff, Jens Seeberg, Lesley Sharp, Bob Simpson, Aja Smith, Olivia Spalletta, Karen-Sue Taussig, Janelle Taylor, Stefan Timmermans, Ayo Wahlberg, and Emily Yates-Doerr. I have also benefited from numerous conversations with my colleagues in the Section for Health Services Research, the Department of Public Health, at the University of Copenhagen. Thank you to Klaus Hoeyer, Allan Krasnik, Henriette Langstrup, Ezio Di Nucci, and Signild Vallgårda. I also thank the members of my current research team, MeInWe—in particular, Ivana Bogicevic, Sara Green, Lotte Groth, Line Hillersdal, Jeanette Knox, Eva Krause, Katharina Ó Cathaoir, Clemence Pinel, and Lea Larsen Skovgaard—for important discussions on welfare state politics.

Thank you to Nancy Chen for coining the title for the book in a café in San Jose, [California], in 2018, and Olivia Spalletta for being such an engaging and educating reader and discussion partner in the final stages of writing. Anne Amalie Wass, one of my student assistants has been an enormous help in putting the bibliography together. It has been a pleasure working with Kim Guinta, my editor at Rutgers University Press, and Lenore Manderson, the series editor. Lenore's enthusiasm and input have been an invaluable support through the whole publication process. I am grateful to the anonymous reviewers of the manuscript who helped me strengthen it and engage more deeply with ethnography and theory. I thank Patricia Piccinini, Tolarno Galleries, and Roslyn Oxley9 Gallery for allowing me to reproduce Picinini's *Undivided* on the book's cover.

Parts of the ethnography and arguments have appeared in articles in *American Ethnologist, BioSocieties, Current Anthropology, Culture, Medicine, and Psychiatry, Critical Public Health, Ethnos, Medical Anthropology, Medical Anthropology Quarterly, Science Technology and Human Values,* and *Social Science and Medicine* and in chapters in *Animal Housing and Human-Animal Relations* (edited by Kristian Bjørkdahl and Tone Druglitrø) and *Biosocial Worlds* (edited by Jens Seeberg, Andreas Roepstorff and Lotte Meinert).

The people who have followed the development of the book most closely are Kåre and our three boys, Eskil, Halfdan, and Asmus. There would be no *Near Human* without their endless patience and inspiration, as well as their efforts to move me away from the computer and remind me of all the other good things in life. My parents, Karen and Peter, were brought up on farms and taught me the fundamentals of Danish agricultural living, the depth of existential questions, and the art of keeping my footing in academic processes. All three areas have given this project a sense of direction and been crucial to its completion. I thank them for their love and dedicate the book to them.

NOTES

PROLOGUE

1. The following discussion of the "just a pig" comment overlaps partly with Svendsen (2017).

INTRODUCTION

1. In already published articles, my coauthors and I have named this pig facility the "Pig Laboratory." When in March 2020 I discussed this term with Professor Per Torp Sangild, who heads the facility, he suggested the term "Newborn Pig Facility." As he said, "a lab is associated with chemistry and analyses, not nurturing (*opfostring*) of animals. Nurturing animals is what characterizes our site. Although we use all the tissue to run analyses, what is unique about our site is our capacity—our facility—to rear weak newborn piglets." His statement captures the emphasis that he and his team put on building up a setting that, in terms of piglets' biology and the care given them, models patients and treatment in the NICU. Thus, I decided to abandon the old name and adopt the new one. Nevertheless, throughout the book I also refer to this site as simply the facility or the lab, and use these terms interchangeably. In particular, I name the experimental site "the lab" when I juxtapose it with "the clinic."

2. I promised all my informants anonymity in my publications. There are a few exceptions, however. The director of the Newborn Pig Facility, Professor Per Torp Sangild, and his closest colleague, Professor Thomas Thymann (who has been central in building up the facility), wanted me to use their real names. I decided to accommodate this wish as they are already public figures. I refer to Per Torp Sangild as "Professor Per" and to Thomas Thymann as "Thomas." Thomas held an associate professorship during my fieldwork years and later became a full professor.

3. In Danish, "*det er vigtigt at se forældrene i øjnene og sige, at et fuldt handicappet liv er vi heller ikke interesseret i.*" A direct translation is, "it is important to look the parents in their eyes and tell them that we are not interested in [saving] a seriously disabled life." Yet in English "not interested in" is dismissive—akin to saying "we would not consider" it. This was not the meaning of the statement as it appeared in the discussion centered on understanding and respecting the parents' perspective. Thus, I changed the wording.

4. The following incident was witnessed by Mie Seest Dam, a graduate student.

5. This engagement with the other is at the crux of the philosopher Emmanuel Lévinas's famous chapter on substitution in *Otherwise than Being* (Lévinas 1974). To Lévinas, the readiness to substitute for the other is integral to becoming a subject. Lévinas compares substitution to the maternal body who bears the other "under her skin" (Lévinas 1974, 109). Consequently, substitution is both the effect of the other in the subject and the ways in which this responsibility is experienced and expressed (Maloney 1997, 61). While I do not embark on a Lévinasian analysis, Lévinas's insights into the intersubjectivity of substitution provide a backdrop for my investigation of the moral and intimate aspects of standing in the position of the other.

6. In her outstanding book on Dolly the sheep, Sarah Franklin points out that the relationship between original and its second is one of asymmetry and that "the fear of being made to

order or copied is one of loss, devaluation, and worthlessness—of being derivative, barren, and unoriginal" (2007, 204). These crucial insights into the relationship between originality and substitution illuminate an ethics of life that tends to evaluate the original as holding absolute worth and the substitute as holding instrumental worth. From this perspective, the use of pigs as models—substitutes—is in itself an expression of their inferiority to humans.

7. For a conceptual framework for understanding animal experiments as sacrifice, see Lynch (1988). For explorations and discussions that extend, refine, and even question this framework, see Haraway (2008), Svendsen and Koch (2013), Lien (2015), Sharp (2019), and chapter 2 in this book.

8. Hinterberger (2018) argues that what should attract the attention of social scientists is not the liminality of these chimeric life-forms, but the ways in which experimental chimeras displace the self-evidence of the human and propel rearticulations of new substantive notions of the human.

9. The concepts of biological and biographical life have affinities with the Greek concepts *zoe* and *bios*, which Giorgio Agamben has revitalized in his work on homo sacer (1998). *Zoe* refers to "bare life," common to all living beings, and *bios* to a qualified life that is protected by law and is a "way of living proper to an individual or group" (Agamben 1998, 10 and 1). This distinction between bare life and qualified life is also a distinction between life and living (Marsland and Prince 2012; Wahlberg 2008) that lies at the very heart of the question "What is a life worth living?"

10. For examples of this perspective, see Barndt (2008); Haraway (2016); Mintz (1986); Tsing (2015); Swanson, Lien, and Ween (2018).

11. To limit the list to the authors who introduced these terms, see Latour on actor network (1987), Woolgar on configurations (1991), Mol on enactment (2002), and Timmermans on script (1996).

12. This section's description of my methodology partly overlaps with Svendsen et al. (2017) and Svendsen et al. (2018).

13. I borrow the phrase "uncanny interface" from Kuan and Grøn's description of the relationship between laboratory studies' third-person perspectives and phenomenological first-person perspectives (2017, 187).

14. Sarah Franklin's work on Dolly the sheep (2007) and its connection to both agriculture and the frontier of human medicine unfolds practices of selection among both humans and sheep, yet this groundbreaking study does not include selection among migrants.

15. Other scholars have challenged the humanist framework of biopolitics in the context of zoos (Chrulew 2013) and science (Friese 2013a, 13–14; Kirk 2016a) and argued for a collapse of the nature-culture dichotomy. This collapse has affinities with the concept of "natureculture," which captures the ways in which the human not only stands in relation to a nonhuman world but also comes into being with this world (Latimer and Miele 2013, 12; see also Haraway 2003).

16. In the years 1875–1877, Denmark produced 41 million kilos of butter and 60 million kilos of pork. In the period 1910–1914 the numbers went up to 112 million kilos of butter and 229 million kilos of pork (Kærgård 2017, 5). In the early twentieth century, as Denmark became the world's leading exporter of pork, especially bacon for the British market, Danish state regulation and state-sponsored control institutions emerged to standardize pig bodies to fit the British market and control the quality of the meat and guarantee disease-free meat (Gjerløff and Jensen 2010).

17. Tiago Saraiva's *Fascist Pigs* unravels the close connections between the modernist political ideology and breeding of livestock to feed "the national body" (2016, 10). Saraiva describes how livestock animals became scientific organisms to serve the nation (2016, 10–11). Although

there was no fascist regime in Denmark, the systematic and nationally coordinated breeding of Danish livestock within a state framework has parallels with modernist ideologies of making the national population thrive on the national soil. In Denmark, nationally coordinated pork production that was organized in a cooperative structure covering the whole chain of production shaped the bodies of pigs through breeding programs, converting pigs to standardized products for export, selling meat of poorer quality on the local market, and reusing the waste products of the pig as animal fodder (Gjerløff and Jensen 2010; Hamann 2006).

18. A Danish textbook for agricultural students explicitly states that the value of every pig in the Danish breeding system refers unambiguously to the economic value of the pig and its offspring for the pig producers and slaughterhouses (Eskildsen and Weber 2018).

19. The Danish Agriculture and Food Council is a powerful organization that includes all the central players in Danish agribusiness. In the organization's own words, "agriculture and food is Denmark's largest competence cluster, employing some 186,000 people and exporting agricultural products, food and equipment to an annual value of around € 20 billion" (Danish Agriculture and Food Council, n.d.). Despite these numbers, agricultural products constituting the top exports in the nineteenth and early twentieth centuries have been overtaken by packaged medicaments such as pharmaceutical products. In 2019, pig meat was Denmark's third most lucrative export item (Observatory of Economic Complexity, n.d.).

20. In Europe, the discussion of animal welfare in production systems was initiated by Ruth Harrison's *Animal Machines: The New Factory Farming Industry* (1964). In Denmark, welfare discussions in relation to the lives of pigs have become particularly prominent since the 1970s and 1980s. Some central issues in this debate are the spaces where the animals live, the animals' possibilities for being stimulated (i.e., enrichment), the conditions in which animals are transported to slaughterhouses, pain related to castration, and the well-being of production sows bred to give birth to some of the largest litters (see chapter 1). Based on an ethnographic study of Danish pig farming, Inger Anneberg and Mette Vaarst state that among pig farmers and welfare legislators there is an expectation that the Danish state will intervene in farming and be responsible for the welfare of animals, even though farmers may be annoyed about the relevant legislation (2018, 101–105). The authors coined the term "the animal welfare state" as a way to explore the mutual shaping of pigs, farmers, and the state (97).

21. Of the cultivated land in Denmark, 80 percent is used for growing fodder for farm animals (Anneberg and Vaarst 2018, 95, note 3).

22. In 2018, only 1.1 per cent of Danish pigs were raised at organic farms that gave them access to the outdoors (Pedersen, Schlægelberger, and Larsen 2018, 1). This means that 98.9 percent of Danish pigs live their whole lives indoors.

23. For this short history of the Royal Veterinary and Agricultural University, I relied on Fritzbøger (2015).

24. "One Health" initiatives craft relationships across disciplines in an effort to understand health links among humans, animals, and the environment. Global networks involving academic and political institutions worldwide promote a 'whole of society' approach to health hazards," viewing health crises and risks as located in the interface between humans, animals, and their environments (One Health Global Network, n.d.). The One Health approach has been central to comparative or translational medicine, which investigates disorders in both humans and animals, including zoonotic diseases. The planetary aspects of health have become increasingly central to One Health movements. In social science, researchers engaged in translational medicine have recently argued for a shift away from targeting an already existing human population to enabling more-than-human "healthy publics" by taking seriously the cultural, social, and environmental relations that make health possible (Hinchliffe et al. 2018).

25. Since the middle of the nineteenth century, the concept of the people has been tightly linked to that of the nation (Hansen 2002; O. Pedersen 2018). Thus, the Danish state-run Lutheran Church is called the Danish People's Church (*Den Danske Folkekirke*), the state-run public school (which covers grades 1–10) is called the People's School (*Folkeskolen*), public health is named people's health (*folkesundhed*), and numerous political parties from the left to the right include "People" in their names—including the Socialist People's Party (*Socialistisk folkeparti*), the Conservative People's Party (*Det konservative folkeparti*), and the Danish People's Party (*Dansk folkeparti*). This tight coupling of the people and the nation can be traced back to the influence of the Danish writer, pastor, philosopher, and politician N.F.S. Grundtvig, whose ideas in the nineteenth century were central to the social movements of enlightenment of the people (*folkeoplysning*), which in turn promoted reciprocal obligation and community education (Jenkins 2011, 44; Einhorn and Logue 2003, 331); as well as the establishment of Danish Folk High Schools (*folkehøjskoler*) and the Danish farmers' coopera- tives (*andelsbevægelse*), which placed a high value on solidarity and equality (H. Jensen 2016, 112–114). Grundtvig put the people at the core of the nation and considered the people the true foundation of Denmark, a construct that the Social Democrats at the beginning of the twentieth century continued to articulate in building up the welfare state. Thus, the slogan of the influential Prime Minister Thorvald Stauning in the 1930s was "Denmark for the People" (Hansen 2002, 60). The tight coupling of people, nation, and state lives on in the widespread use and positive connotations of "the people" in public discourse.

26. In the 1990s, new public management reforms tightened access to welfare support by reducing the duration of unemployment benefits and introducing stricter requirements for being available to participate in the labor market (Larsen and Andersen 2009). Neoliberal reforms also introduced economic incentives to increase the productivity of health care, for instance by case-based payments in the hospital sector, and a stronger focus on patient choice, for instance by providing access to free prenatal screening for all pregnant women regardless of age. Despite these reforms to increase the labor supply and improve performance and efficiency in health care, neoliberal influences in Danish politics have not resulted in the retrenchment of welfare state institutions. Today, democratically elected bodies have retained control of central societal fields such as social security, health care, and education, and an all-embracing social welfare system is taken for granted as the preferred principle of societal organization supported by the population and all parties in the Danish Parliament.

27. In 2006, the Fertility Law was amended to provide women ages 18–40 with access to three cycles of IVF and insemination procedures subsidized by the state, up to the birth of one child. The law, which in Danish is called *Lov om kunstig befrugtning* (Law on artificial insemination), regulates access to many different forms of assistive reproductive technolo- gies, and it is periodically updated to incorporate advances in reproductive medicine. The law reflects Denmark's liberal approach to what makes a family. This is also expressed in a report from Statistics Denmark, the central authority on Danish statistics, which lists thirty-seven different family types in Denmark (2018, 31). Access to IVF in public clinics is conditional on the patient's being a resident or having a work permit in the country, and thus asylum seekers are excluded. In addition to IVF clinics in the public health care system, Denmark has a num- ber of private IVF clinics. Here, waiting lists are often shorter than at the public clinics (at least in the Copenhagen area), and there is no restriction on the number of children. Thus, couples or single women who already have one child need to pay for IVF treatment for subse- quent children in private clinics.

28. For these numbers, I relied on Professor of Prenatal Diagnostics Ida Vogel's description in *Den Store Danske* (Vogel 2017) and Spalletta (2021).

29. As principal investigator of the LifeWorth project and partner in the NEOMUNE platform, I embarked on a thoroughly collaborative way of doing ethnography and writing papers. While the three graduate students and the associate professor mentioned in the text conducted fieldwork in specific ethnographic sites, I participated in some of the fieldwork in each site, supervised team members by acting as the active last author on publications, and invited them to be coauthors of publications where I was the first author. Through monthly meetings, I steered the work of bringing the studies together to focus on the worth of lives. In experimenting with this collaborative way of working, I drew on the experiences of collaborative work employed in the science fields we investigated.

30. The ethnographic material on which this book is based covers eleven weeks of following experimental studies in the Newborn Pig Facility and related sites (carried out by Mie Seest Dam and me between 2009 and 2014) and twenty weeks of fieldwork following clinicians in their daily work in the human NICU (carried out by Laura Emdal Navne and me between 2010 and 2014); participation in numerous scientific seminars related to the experimental pig studies, including NEOMUNE symposia; conducting twenty-five interviews with researchers connected to animal-based experimental science, one interview with the head of the company producing cow colostrum for NICUs, one interview with the Danish owner of a large piggery, one interview with the head of a Danish zoo that housed rehabilitated research monkeys, two interviews with researchers conducting research on monkeys in research sites in Asia, five interviews with representatives of Danish animal welfare organizations or the Danish pharmaceutical industry, twenty interviews with staff members in the NICU, and two interviews with employees of the Danish Health Authority. Most of these interviews were carried out by one or two members of the LifeWorth team (Lene, Mie, Laura, Iben, Anja, and me) or one or two members of the Pig Project team (Lene; Vibeke Pihl, a graduate student; and me). In addition, Jeanette Knox, another graduate student, and I carried out two focus groups with NICU staff members in 2013; Mie interviewed fourteen parents about their experiences and expectations in relation to the feeding of their premature children; and Mie and I supervised two master's degree students, Julie Borring and Ditte Hansen, who conducted a study of the human milk bank that provides donor milk to NICUs in Eastern Denmark and experiments in the Newborn Pig Facility. In chapter 1, I draw on some of this material. The book also rests on the foundation of my twenty years of researching Danish health care practices, including studies on cancer genetics (1999–2004), embryonic stem cell research (2004–2008), pharmacogenomics (2006–2009), dementia care together with Iben (2013–2019), and precision medicine (2017–2022).

In the Newborn Pig Facility, I stood next to the researchers during the cesarean sections and delivery of the piglets; I followed the researchers in attending to the piglets, feeding them, doing tests on them, and eventually killing them; and I went into the laboratories where samples were prepared and analyzed. I became acquainted with the researchers' meticulous care for the piglets, their strong and unique team spirit, their admirable commitment to turning the piglets into scientific samples with the hope of creating new knowledge and improving the health of infants in the clinic, and the concurrent transformation of first-year graduate students into full-fledged scientists.

In the human NICU, I entered the conference room and listened to medical rounds, and I was present when clinicians gave information about premature birth and treatment possibilities to couples who expected to have an early delivery. I observed doctors treating infants, looking up medical records in the computer, engaging in small talk with parents at their infant's bedside, and informing them behind closed doors about their child's situation. I also followed the nurses who spent many hours next to the infants and worked closely with their parents.

31. Etho-ethnography combines ethology and ethnography, thus expanding culture beyond the human world (Buller 2014).

CHAPTER 1 FEEDING

1. This specific ethnographic example of Thomas referring to Mie as *madmor* also appears in Dam et al. (2017).

2. The researchers would also use the term "the big NEOMUNE family" when referring to collaboration between the laboratory and the clinic in the NEOMUNE research platform and when taking photos of the entire group of about sixty people at conference sites.

3. All present breeds of swine are related to the wild boar, *Sus scrofa,* which was domesticated in Asia around 8500 B.C. and brought to Europe by 4500 B.C. DNA analysis suggests that pig domestication was an ongoing process and largely took place by breeding domesticated animals with local wild boars (Caliebe et al. 2017). The use of pigs as model animals is known from "ancient Greece, where Erasistratus (304–250 B.C.) used them to investigate the mechanics of breathing. In Rome, Galen (130–200 A.D.) used them to demonstrate blood circulation" (U.S. Department of Health and Human Services, n.d.).

4. In Danish maternity wards, colostrum is referred to as precious drops, while in the United States, it is referred to as liquid gold. Both terms signal that the liquid is invaluable for the newborn baby.

5. In the pilot study in the Danish NICU, standard feeding included mother's milk supplemented by human donor milk if mother's milk was not available in sufficient amounts, and cow colostrum replaced human donor milk. In the pilot study in the Chinese NICU, standard feeding included mother's milk supplemented by infant formula if mother's milk was not sufficiently available, and cow colostrum replaced infant formula (see also Li et al. 2017).

6. This couple was interviewed by Mie and Sandra M. Juhl, a graduate student, as part of preparing a larger randomized study to test the safety and efficacy outcomes in preterm infants.

7. In the field of kinship in anthropology, David Schneider's *American Kinship* (1980) provided a turning point in laying bare the ways in which biological facts were privileged in Western ways of thinking. His scholarship powerfully reveals how indigenous Euro-American kinship thinking was imported into the anthropological analysis (see, e.g., Schneider 1984, 174–175). His critique marginalized the topic of kinship in anthropology in the 1960s and 1970s. In the 1990s, kinship studies were revived, concurrently with the development of new reproductive and genetic technologies (see, e.g., Franklin 1997; J. Edwards et al. 1999; Konrad 2005; Strathern 1992a, 1992b). Carsten's concept of relatedness belongs to this era and has been crucial in challenging a universal distinction between biology and social relations and paving the way for a processual perspective on kinship. Central to the concept of relatedness is an orientation toward actions and ideas about connection and disconnection. She suggests directing analytical attention toward the components of kinship (e.g., procreation, blood, food, coresidence, and shared memory) and the process of constructing kinship (Carsten 1995, 1997).

8. Schneider's humorous description of his conversations with the Yap people about the relationship between coitus and pregnancy is illustrative of the Western idea about universal biological continuity between humans and animals and its limits in other parts of the world. While the Yap agreed with Schneider that a castrated pig cannot make a sow pregnant, they insisted that coitus among humans does not result in pregnancy. Instead, ancestral ghosts get the spirit to bestow pregnancy. To Schneider, Yap statements about pigs and humans were logically inconsistent, and he described the contradiction to the Yap. They did not acknowl-

edge the contradiction until suddenly a man saw Schneider's problem and responded, "But people are not pigs" (Schneider 1980, 128).

9. Gunner asked me to use the real name for the company and for him and Betina, his employee whose work practices I followed.

10. In 1992, selection for litter size was initiated in Danish pig production (Rutherford et al. 2011, 24; Haugegaard 2006, 10). Between 1996 and 2009 the number of piglets born in Denmark increased 33 percent, while the number of weaned piglets increased only 23 percent. The numbers illustrate that "a significant proportion of the selection effort . . . has gone towards producing stillborn piglets" (Rutherford et al. 2011, 28), yet the selection effort resulted in more pigs for the pig farmers and constituted an economic advantage. In 2004 the selection criterion was changed from number of born piglets to the number of piglets living at day five. This resulted in a reduction of piglet mortality from 24.2 percent in 2009 to 21.3 percent in 2016, yet in 2017 the mortality rate had risen to 21.7 percent (Høyer, 2018).

11. "*Overdimensionerede kuld fører til milliondød blandt smågrise* [Oversized litters cause millions of deaths in piglets]," *Politiken*, May 18, 2010. See also *Fastholder kritik* [Maintains critique]," *Effektivt Landbrug*, May 20, 2010; "*Høj dødelighed blandt pattegrise er ikke i strid med loven* [High mortality rate among piglets is not against the law]," *Effektivt Landbrug*, June 10, 2010.

12. The first systematic breeding of Danish Landrace pigs and Yorkshire pigs in Denmark was initiated in 1895. In Denmark, pig breeding is centralized in one organization, DanBred, a subsidiary of the Danish Agriculture and Food Council. In DanBred's descriptions of pig breeding, the concepts of production traits, genetic improvement, breeding objectives, and adaptation of those objectives to economic conditions underpin the understanding of the pig as clay in the hands of the industry. Every pig at a breeding farm has a eleven-digit number, and every week its value is assessed based on the breeding goals. Only the animals with the highest numbers will live and continue to be part of the breeding system; animals with lower numbers will be killed (Eskildsen and Weber 2018, 186–193). The current breeding objectives (defined in 2015) are growth, utilization of fodder, lean meat percentage, leg strength, slaughter loss (the loss of usable meat due for instance to abscesses, disease, bruises), longevity of sows, and reduced piglet mortality (DanBred 2018). The breeding practices use genomic selection that draws on the swine genome, which is the result of a global collaborative effort among researchers in China (at the Beijing Genomics Institute), Denmark (at Aarhus and Copenhagen Universities), and elsewhere.

13. These dead bodies entered the welfare state collectivity in other ways. In Denmark, discarded animal bodies and parts are reused in a number of ways. For example, in 2008, the Danish company Daka opened a new factory that converts dead animal bodies to bio fuel used in public transportation.

14. In Denmark, it is common to change the names and responsibilities of ministries to reflect central political agendas. Thus through time, ministerial responsibility for the field of food and agriculture has belonged to ministries of different names. To avoid confusion, I will use the generic terms "Ministry of Food and Agriculture" and "minister of food and agriculture."

15. Henrik Høegh, from the center-right party, was the minister of food at the time. He is a farmer and has held a number of influential positions in agricultural associations that are now part of the Danish agriculture and food council. In response to the news about the high percentage of newborn piglets dying in the farrowing pens, Høegh and spokespeople from other political parties stated that the death rates were unacceptable and took political action by initiating a thorough and impartial investigation of the situation. In a response to the criticism, the Danish Agriculture and Food Council used the much higher mortality rates among wild boar and free-range pigs to argue that conditions in the farrowing pens were good compared to those in nature. The Animal Protection Society replied that when humans keep animals, it is not nature that rules, but the animal protection act (Dyrenes beskyttelse June 02, 2010). While one side naturalized piglet mortality, the other depicted death as a human responsibility.

16. In Danish, *"Folketinget bør gribe ind over for svineavlen, hvis landmændene ikke selv gør noget"* (quoted in Vibeke Rask Grøn, *"K overvejer politisk indgreb mod svineavl* [K considers political intervention over pig breeding]," May 18, 2010, *dr.dk*, accessed April 12, 2021, https://www.dr.dk/nyheder/indland/k-overvejer-politisk-indgreb-mod-svineavl).

17. In Danish, *"problematisk at vi ser en stigning i dødeligheden"* (quoted in*"Høj dødelighed blandt pattegrise er ikke i strid med loven* [High mortality among piglets is not against the law]," June 10, 2010, *Effektivt Landbrug,* accessed April 12, 2021, https://effektivtlandbrug.land brugnet.dk/artikler/arkiv/25792/hoej-doedelighed-blandt-pattegrise-er-ikke-i-strid-med -loven.aspx).

18. *"Danske svineavlere indklaget for EU* [Complaints about Danish pig farmers filed with the EU]," May 19, 2010.

19. Quoted in T. Jensen (2013, 133).

20. The links between the history of agricultural innovation and the development of life science are masterfully analyzed by Sarah Franklin, who describes the ways in which Dolly the sheep was a result of "comingl[ing] lineages of science and industry with those of agriculture and medicine" (2007, 154).

21. The old-fashioned piggy bank containing spare coins saved over a longer period of time epitomizes this process. Such ceramic banks did not have the now common rubber plug on the underside and had to be smashed to obtain the saved money. The same is true of the laboratory pig: its death at the end of the experiment is a prerequisite for transforming cow colostrum into human nutrition.

22. In *Animal Parasites and Messmates,* Pierre van Beneden (1876) introduced the term "commensal associates" to describe animals that ate the waste food of other animals (like carcass eaters). In the case of the relationship between the preindustrial pig and the human, the two related meanings (sharing a meal and eating waste food) coexist.

23. Theories of waste and value show that disposal is not about making something disappear, but about placing an object in a transient category and facilitating its possible reevaluation. In his theory of rubbish, the anthropologist Michael Thompson argues that classifying an object as rubbish has the potential to transfer it from the transient category of waste to a durable category, thereby reevaluating a waste object (1979, 8–9, 44–45). For further discussions of disposal and waste and the potential for reevaluation, see Kevin Hetherington (2004); Gjødsbøl, Koch, and Svendsen (2017); Svendsen (2011); C. Thompson (2005); Waldby and Mitchell (2006).

24. In 2018, 22,000 bull calves were killed at birth in Denmark (*"Kan man undgå at kalve aflives ved fødslen?* [Can calf deaths at birth be avoided?]," n.d., *Mejeri.dk*). One farmer told me that the alternative to killing the bull calves at birth is to send them to the Netherlands to be fostered as "milk calves," which he described as "putting them behind bars in a small cage and only feeding them milk for eighteen months to generate a particularly tender meat." To him, killing bull calves at birth was much more ethically acceptable than giving them the compromised welfare of "milk calves."

25. Colostrum as animal fodder is Biofiber's main product and the source of its most stable and largest income. The company's investment in colostrum for humans and its articulation of this product as of greater significance than animal fodder indicate the status and potential value attached to producing nutrition for preterm infants.

26. See Sangild and colleagues (2014) for a detailed description of the preterm pig as a translational model in pediatric gastroenterology.

27. Similarly, Emily Yates-Doerr reminds us that "families can be formed from difference, not merely from resemblance" (2015, 316).

28. Danish NICUs are world leaders in including parents as well as doctors in decision making about children and involving parents in the care for their child (Greisen and Henriksen 2018; Solberg 2018).

29. The Danish Health Authority (2013) puts a great emphasis on breast-feeding and recommends exclusive breast-feeding up to the age of approximately six months.

30. The following example was experienced by Mie and also appears in Svendsen and colleagues (2017).

31. These interviews were carried out by Dam and Juhl as part of preparing the NEOMUNE randomized controlled pilot study based on results from the pig studies. The interviews aimed at identifying the parents' and pregnant women's experiences and expectations in relation to feeding a premature infant. All interviews took place at the bedside or in an office in the NICU. Some of the following interview quotes and analyses also appear in Dam et al. (2017).

32. The quotes in this paragraph come from a study on the donation and processing of human donor milk (Borring and Hansen 2017) carried out by two master's degree students I supervised in 2016–2017. The study's results were later published as Borring et al. (2018).

33. See Katherine Carroll's study (2016) of NICU mothers' ambiguity about human donor milk and Kristin Wilson's study (2018) of exceptional breast-feeders in the United States. Wilson explores the societal norms of breast-feeding as the essence of motherhood, thus providing a backdrop for the Danish NICU mothers' unease with human donor milk. As her ethnography powerfully demonstrates, the intimacy involved in sharing breast milk may give way to highly innovative and positive forms of relatedness, yet it may also create experiences of jealousy.

34. This quote and the next come from a study on the donation and processing of human donor milk (Borring and Hansen 2017).

35. In his book about metabolic disease in India, Solomon uses this phrase in connection to the always lurking risk of polluted foods brought from the market into the home and cooked by housewives (2016, 119). Here I extend the kinship between those who cook and those who eat to include the animals from which the substance originates.

CHAPTER 2 KILLING

1. In anthropological studies of sacrifice, substitution plays a central role as violence is moved from the original to the substitute, executed in a demarcated time and space, and legitimized and made sacred by the anticipation of a future return (Birke 2003; Bloch 1992; Durkheim 1915; Girard 1977; Govindrajan 2015; Haraway 1997; Hubert and Mauss 1968; Smith and Doniger 1989; Willerslev 2009).

2. In her phenomenological examination of physical suffering, Elaine Scarry argues that what distinguishes unmaking and making is not the difference between the weapon and the tool, but the surface on which it falls. While the axe that cuts through the back of a wolf is a weapon, the axe that cuts through a tree is a tool. This is so because the weapon acts on a sentient surface and the tool acts on a nonsentient surface (Scarry 1985, 173–174). Similarly, we may see the experiment simultaneously as a weapon that unmakes piglet life by imposing suffering and death on the animals and as a tool that remakes piglet life by turning the piglets into tissue samples (see Svendsen and Koch 2013).

3. Examples of individual care for the piglets include removing air from the abdomen, read-justing catheters, and carrying out cardiopulmonary resuscitation.

4. This interview quote also appears in Svendsen and colleagues (2018).

5. This interview quote also appears in Svendsen and Koch (2013).

6. This resonates with Emmanuel Lévinas's proposition that substituting for another involves not only becoming the host for another, but also corporeal hostage of the other (1974). In the case of Marie and the piglet, Marie was not only hosting the pig in her scientific household, she was also "punctualized by a demanding relation" (Latimer 2013, 97; see also Munro 2004) and called on to take care of the piglet.

7. The principles of replacement, reduction, and refinement have constituted the dominant ethical framework for animal research. Replacement refers to replacing animal models with alternatives. Reduction refers to reducing the number of animals to a minimum. Refinement refers to developing methods that reduce the suffering of animals to the greatest possible extent (W. Russell et al. 1959).

8. This interview quote also appears in Svendsen and Koch (2013).

9. In the Newborn Pig Facility, standardization was not questioned. Rather, individual treat-ment was integrated into the standardized setup, and the relationship between standardiza-tion and individualization was referred to as a "balancing act" (Dam and Svendsen 2018, 364). For instance, researchers provided individual care in the form of blowing air into the lungs of a newborn piglet to optimize its chances of survival, yet they were more reluctant to change the dosing of nutrition, which they saw as essential to standardization.

10. The following analysis of the group discussion also appears in Svendsen (2020).

11. The following episode happened during Mie's fieldwork and is also described in Svend-sen and colleagues (2017).

12. This section on patientization is based on Dam and Svendsen (2018).

13. Mie experienced this episode in 2013 (see also Dam and Svendsen 2018).

14. The following description also appears in Svendsen and Koch (2013).

15. This quote also appears in Dam et al. (2017).

16. The example of Julie and Röntgen is described in Svendsen (2016).

17. This example also appears in Svendsen and Koch (2013).

18. The concept of the uncanny refers both to the familiar and to what is concealed and kept out of sight, which according to Sigmund Freud signifies the familiar that has been repressed (1978, 224–225).

19. See Koch and Svendsen (2015, 2016). The following builds on Koch and Svendsen (2015).

20. The oldest of the cages were 0.70 by 0.70 by 0.85 meters in size.

21. The new directive was adopted in September 2010 (European Union 2010). Two years earlier, in 2008, Spain granted legal rights to great apes.

22. Jensen and Mathiessen, "Novo: Forsøgsaber skal slippes fri [Novo: Research monkeys need to be liberated]," Ingeniøren, June 20, 2003.

CHAPTER 3 TREATING

1. The following discussion of guidelines as a political act of letting infants in and out of soci-ety overlaps with Navne and Svendsen (2019).

2. This guideline was in preparation during my first period of fieldwork and in use during Laura Emdal Navne's fieldwork.

3. This politics of life has support in the general population. A study based on responses to a questionnaire from seven hundred randomly selected Danes ages 19–44 concluded that "there was an almost uniform agreement [among respondents] that not all [NICU] infants

ought to be treated no matter how serious the condition" (Norup 1998, 205) and that "parental attitude towards treatment is considered important by many" (206). For a historical perspective on policies and public discussion about the treatment of preterm infants in Denmark, see Greisen and Henriksen (2018).

4. In Denmark, the state-funded Lutheran church (the Danish People's Church) is very liberal, and the great majority of church spokespeople support abortion rights.

5. See Gammeltoft and Wahlberg (2014) for an outline of selective reproduction through time and space. Central anthropological studies of selective reproduction include Nancy Scheper-Hughes's work on high infant mortality as a result of extreme economic deprivation in a shanty town in Brazil in the 1980s (1992); Rupert Stasch's study of abandonment of newborn infants in past practices in Papua New Guinea (2009); Lynn Morgan's work on bottled fetuses in reproductive science at the beginning of the twentieth century in Baltimore, Maryland (2009); and Tine Gammeltoft's study of the moral dilemmas facing pregnant women in Vietnam who late in their pregnancy learned about fetal abnormalities (2014). Eugenics is another form of selection closely linked to biomedicine (Koch 2014). In the late twentieth and early twenty-first century, biomedicine has provided a range of new possibilities for making decisions about "which gametes to fertilize, which embryos to implant or which fetuses to abort" (Wahlberg and Gammeltoft 2018, 1), and anthropologists are increasingly studying these processes (e.g., Bharadwaj 2008; Franklin 2012; Franklin and Roberts 2006; Gammeltoft 2014; Rapp 1999; Roberts 2007; Wahlberg 2018). What unites the studies of selective reproduction outside biomedicine with studies of selective reproduction by way of biotechnological manipulation is their investigation of the social, economic, and political contexts of childbearing interventions. I lean on this focus in the following discussion, yet I expand the context by moving across the human-animal divide—viewing selective reproduction as not only a human affair, but as practiced among animals in livestock and life science.

6. In this case, the couple's IVF treatment was funded by the state, yet five weeks after the birth of the child, the social authorities removed the child from the parents as they were not considered able to take care of it ("*Først fik de fertilitetsbehandling - så blev barnet tvangsfjernet* [First they received fertility treatment—then the child was removed by the social authorities]," TV2/Fyn, May 17, 2010). The fertility doctors involved were heavily criticized by the Minister of Health, and the Fertility Law as revised in 2010 instructs fertility clinics to contact other professionals (such as the couple's general practitioner) and/or social authorities in case of any doubt about a couple's ability to parent. The new law stated: "The parents or the single woman need to consent to the involvement of other professionals in the assessment of parental ability. If the parents or the single woman do not consent, the fertility doctor must decline from initiating treatment" (*Med parrets eller den enlige kvindes samtykke kan den praktiserende læge eller sociale myndigheder således inddrages ved vurderingen af omsorgsevnen. Ved manglende samtykke skal lægen afvise at indlede behandling med kunstig befrugtning*) (Fertility Law 2010, Section 2.1).

7. The guidelines cited in the text were in use during my fieldwork in the NICU. They have been revised since. The most recent guidelines refer to a number of initiatives aimed at supporting pregnant women who suffer from social or psychological problems. These guidelines also recommend that pregnant women who suffer from drug addiction be informed about the possibility of abortion if they are in the early stages of pregnancy (Danish Health Authority 2013, 65).

8. A shorter version of this case is presented in Svendsen (2015).

9. This interview quote also appears in Navne and Svendsen (2019).

10. In her ethnography of Black American families with children who had serious chronic diseases, Cheryl Mattingly calls this "dramatic time" (2010, 163), a linear temporality in which

it is uncertain what will happen next. In the context of the NICU, such a time has been described as a temporality in which "past, present, and future are subsequent stages in a development marked by progression" (Mesman 2008, 140).

11. This quote and analysis also appear in Svendsen et al. (2018).

12. The case of Tobias is also described in Svendsen (2015).

13. This quote and the following analysis of premature life as being at the margins of time and society overlaps with Svendsen et al. (2018).

14. It should be noted, though, that in some situations the word was not only an institutional language used among doctors. It was also shared with parents when clinicians invited them to have a *"mors* conversation" to talk through the process leading to the death of their child.

15. Thank you to Lillian Prueher for having brought the dynamics of storage to my attention.

16. See Navne and Svendsen (2018) for a detailed analysis of this case.

17. The following analysis of resource discussions in the NICU overlaps with Svendsen (2020).

18. This separation between human life and economy echoes the common view that the value of the human body should be kept separate from monetary transactions (Felt et al. 2009; Hoeyer 2005; Svendsen 2007). With the concept of unknowing, I refer not to a lack of knowledge but to a form of knowledge—in this case, about economic resources—that is out of place and therefore may make it difficult for organizations to function and pursue their goals (Geissler 2013; Mathews 2011).

19. The concepts of the deserving and undeserving poor have been part of social politics in Denmark since the late nineteenth century (Kolstrup 2011).

20. The basic arguments for this group of eugenic laws were utilitarian and aimed at protecting the national economy as well as the hereditary and moral health of the nation. Although the laws legalized forced sterilization, the expectation was that the people who were targeted would eventually consent to the procedure (Koch 2014, 107). In explaining the need for selection, Victor Pürshel, a conservative politician, said: "In earlier times when feebleminded women gave birth, it often resulted in child murder. . . . Today, everything women give birth to is kept alive and this means that society needs to execute the selection" (quoted, 116).

21. In Danish, *"Afbrydelse af svangerskab på grund af frygten for, at afkommet skal arve legemlige eller sjælelige sygdomme, psykiske abnormaliteter, kriminelle tilbøjeligheder o.lign fra forældrene"* (quoted in Koch 2014, 137).

22. In Danish, *"Ethvert menneskeligt væsen skal have ret til den lykkeligst mulige tilværelse, og skal om fornødent beskyttes og plejes. Kun i en henseende må samfundet være på sin post: med hensyn til forplantningen. . . . Vi behandler undermåleren med al omsigt og kærlighed men forbyder ham blot til gengæld at forplante sig"* (quoted in Koch 2014, 43–44).

23. For descriptions of what was considered excessive sexuality and loathsome fertility, see Koch (2014, 110).

24. While policies as practices of substitution articulate a moral stance on who to substitute for and who to exclude, they generate a cascade of other substitution practices when they are interpreted in specific spaces and situations. Similar to what we have seen in the NICU and the Newborn Pig Facility, where professionals make decisions about life and death, in the 1930s clinicians and state agents in Danish municipalities were the ones to interpret the reforms and make decisions about who to support and who not to support—thus engaging in practices of substitution. Consequently, I do not make the traditional distinction between policies as discourses and daily interactions as social practices. Instead, I conceptualize policies as social practices being enacted and intervening in the world. With this approach, both policies and daily practices may be conceptualized as practices of substitution.

25. In the beginning of the twentieth century, Wilhelm Johannsen, a Danish scientist, developed a genetic theory and the concept of "pure lines" (Roll-Hansen 2005; Müller-Wille 2008). The emerging science of heredity was part of a new modernity concerned with social and economic progress. This implied denouncing tradition and inheritance, concepts that belonged to the past (Müller-Wille 2008).

26. Germany introduced its first eugenic legislation in 1933.

27. Roger Griffin (2007) argues that at the core of fascist ideologies is a drive for a new birth of society, an alternative modernity. Similarly, studies on eugenics movements emphasize their obsession with the future (Koch 2014; Müller-Wille 2008; Murphy 2017). In her study on the economization of life, Michelle Murphy argues that the 1930s eugenics movement in the United States identified biology and heredity as a framework of differentiation, whereas the subsequent cold-war logic of economic development calculated "the differential worth of racialized bodies in terms of their contribution to future economic productivity" (Murphy 2017, 11–12). In the Danish context, the two frameworks seem to have coexisted, as the problem with the unfit was not so much one of racial biological inferiority as it was their expected low contribution to future economic productivity. The aim of the Danish eugenics movement was to establish a new order and create a morally, economically, and socially sustainable future (Koch 2014, 41–45).

28. The public debate preceding the legalization did not discuss heredity (as was the case in the 1930s) but saw the social situation of the mother as the relevant criterion for ending lives not yet born. The dominant argument was that if the situation of the mother was not optimal, she should have the possibility to make a responsible choice of abortion, as the mother's situation might worsen with the addition of a child, and unwanted children may have poor lives (Nexø 2009).

29. In Danish, "*Den prænatale diagnostik vil derfor kunne få stor betydning for samfundet ved at forhindre fødsel af børn med livsvarigt handicap, der vil have behov for gentagne hospitaliseringer eller livslangt ophold på institution. Ved denne diagnostik kan store menneskelige tragedier forhindres. Når dertil kommer, at en del af den prænatale diagnostik kan udføres således, at de samfundsmæssige besparelser set ud fra et cost-benefit synspunkt balancerer med eller overstiger det offentliges udgifter i forbindelse med de pågældende undersøgelsers foretagelse, finder udvalget, at det offentlige vil opnå en meget stor fordel ved at prioritere denne prænatale diagnostik højt i fremtidens sundhedspolitik*" (Danish Ministry of Interior Affairs 1977, 37).

30. The age criterion of thirty-five also reflects the aim of cost-effectiveness, as the risk of a fetus's having Down syndrome increases with the age of the woman.

31. While Danish reproductive policies in the 1930s included the use of force to avoid the creation of unfit lives, policies in the 1970s relied to a greater extent on women's taking the responsibility for terminating pregnancies and embracing the public health interventions of the welfare state. From a Foucauldian perspective, these processes of self-governance have been powerfully described as government through freedom (see, e.g., Rose 1999; Vallgårda 2003).

32. All over Europe and in the United States, IVF brought about a reflection on the dominant cultural ideas about reproduction (Strathern 1992b) and created an ethical maelstrom of questions about the possibilities for manipulating, designing, and cloning human beings (Jonsen 1998, 305–306), followed by questions about how to regulate these possibilities. In the United States and Britain, committees were established to discuss the implications of the new technologies, and reports were published (U.S. President's Commission for the Study of Ethical Problems in Medicine and Biomedical and Behavioral Research 1982; U.K. Department of Health and Social Security 1984). The Danish report took a moderately positive stance toward including IVF technologies in public health (Danish Ministry of Interior

Affairs 1984). Two years later, IVF was approved as a state-financed treatment in public hospitals in Denmark (Mohr and Koch 2016, 91).

33. The report argued that cost-benefit calculations should not lead to a view on disabled people as solely an unnecessary "expense for society," as such a view would "threaten the investments of social political ambitions for many years" (Danish Ministry of Interior Affairs 1984, 47).

34. These guidelines ensure that every pregnant woman is offered a prenatal risk assessment before gestation week twelve (Danish Health Authority 2004). The risk assessment comes in the form of a risk figure for Down syndrome.

35. Denmark was the first country in the world to make nuchal translucency scans available to all pregnant women regardless of age. Maternal serum markers, the scan, and the woman's age-related risk are combined to calculate an overall risk figure. According to the guidelines, only women with a risk of 1 in 300 (or 0.3 percent) have access to invasive testing (Danish Health Authority 2017). As the risk of inducing a miscarriage of a nonaffected fetus is 1 in 100 (1.0 percent), it might be speculated that the Danish health authorities consider a child with Down syndrome to be a higher risk for society than the risk of miscarrying a healthy fetus for the individual woman (Schwennesen, Svendsen, and Koch 2010, 210). In March 2017, the noninvasive prenatal test was introduced in Danish health care for women with a high risk of giving birth to a child with a chromosomal abnormality. This is a DNA test that uses maternal blood to screen pregnancies for trisomy 21 (Down syndrome), trisomy 18 (Edwards syndrome) and trisomy 13 (Patau syndrome). The test also determines the gender of the fetus. It does not carry any risk of abortion.

CHAPTER 4 METABOLIZING

1. In the introduction to *The Biometric Border World*, Karen Fog Olwig and her colleagues write that "'assemblage' . . . makes it possible to avoid conceptualizing the border world as a rational, coherent, intentionally built well-oiled whole while at the same time enabling us to detect how it is composed of partially connected elements, as well as correlated coercive and conflicting forces" (2020, viii). My investigation of the various imaginations of society that come to the fore in the entry and exit processes that constitute the border as a sociospatial assemblage is inspired by this approach.

2. The term human migrant covers a variety of people traveling across borders: refugees fleeing armed conflict, people moving to improve their lives, asylum seekers, undocumented foreigners, and people who have citizenship yet in public discourse are categorized as in need of integration. By using the term "human immigrants," I do not wish to naturalize their otherness to society. Rather, I aim to uncover the conceptions and imaginaries about society that come to the fore in boundary maintenance and social exclusion. In the following discussion, I use the terms "migrants," "labor migrants," and "refugees" to uncover the categorizations of various policies and spokespeople.

3. Denmark is the country that produces most pigs per capita, yet China is the world's largest producer and consumer of pork. China consumes the same amount of pork as the rest of the world does. In Chinese, the pig is a symbol of fertility and prosperity: the traditional radical for "home" is a pig under a roof. Since the 1970s, the industrialization and urbanization of China have created a middle class whose fortunes and spending powers have grown concurrently with China's rise.

4. Bent Højgaard Sørensen, *"Tulippølser vælter den kinesiske mur* [Tulip sausages topple the Great Wall of China]," *Berlingske Tidende*, November 25, 2013.

5. Pia Guld Munksgaard, "*I Kina spiser de. . . . danske pølser,*" Danish National Radio and Television, April 17, 2014, https://www.dr.dk/nyheder/politik/i-kina-spiser-de-danske-poelser.

6. Quoted in "*Kinesiske forbrugere skal spise mere dansk gris* [Chinese consumers should eat more Danish pork]," *Landbrug og Fødevarer,* May 16, 2018.

7. Lars Attrup, "*Svinepest i Asien giver jackpot: Eksportrekord og milliardregn over landbruget* [Hitting the jackpot due to swine fever in Asia: New export record is a billion-crown shower for farming]," *Jyllandsposten,* June 12, 2019; Astrid Sofie Sturlason, "*Kina ramt af fatal svinepest: Det er en 'gamechanger'* [Fatal swine fever in China: It's a 'game changer']," *Berlingske Tidende,* April 23, 2019.

8. March 2020, five hundred infants had been fed cow colostrum as part of NEOMUNE and NEOCOL protocols in ten Chinese and eight Danish NICUs, collectively.

9. In social science, the contribution of research subjects in transnational clinical trials has been conceptualized as value-producing labor (see, e.g., Rajan 2007; Cooper and Waldby 2014), and trials moved offshore have been described as epistemic infrastructures that economize life and categorize lives into those more or less worthy of living (Murphy 2017). While the NEOMUNE and NEOCOL studies in China do exemplify the transnational production of knowledge and the intervention in precarious (infant) populations for the sake of generating both health and wealth, these specific trials also complicate the simple picture of a Western exploiter and an Eastern population that is being exploited. In NEOMUNE and NEOCOL, it was not the outsourcing of risk, but access to a larger population that was at the crux of the collaboration. Yet what the NEOMUNE and NEOCOL studies in both Denmark and China illustrate is how building knowledge infrastructures and creating study populations govern life in ways that link it to national economies. Michelle Murphy (2017) describes this as the entanglement between reproduction, experiment, and economy.

10. The NEOMUNE randomized controlled pilot study, which I described in chapter 1, included Danish and Chinese infants in the same cohort. Based on the knowledge of and experience with the Chinese setting gained through the NEOMUNE years, the NEOCOL clinical studies were designed differently. One study was to be conducted among children who had access to mother's milk. At the time of the meeting in Shenzhen, this study was envisioned to include six NICUs in Denmark and two in China where mothers can enter the hospital and turn in breast milk for their child. Another study was to be conducted among children in ten hospitals in China who had no access to their mother's milk. Due to the big differences between Danish and Chinese treatment practices, the team ended up designing three studies: one for eight Danish NICUs where mother's milk and human donor milk were available (two more than originally planned); one for the two Chinese NICUs that offered human donor milk; and one for the remaining ten Chinese NICUs where human donor milk was not an option.

11. In Denmark, 60 percent of the land area is cultivated (Holmstrup et al. 2018, 6) and 80 percent of the cultivated land is used for growing fodder for farm animals (Anneberg and Vaarst 2018, 95, note 3).

12. Christian Erin-Madsen, "*Sådan hænger danske grise sammen med misdannede børn i Argentina* [This is the connection between Danish pigs and malformed children in Argentina]," *DanWatch,* April 9, 2019.

13. Martin Bahn, "*Ny rapport: Skov blive ryddet for at skaffe foder til danske svin* [New report: Fodder for Danish pigs causes deforestation]," *Information,* October 2, 2018; Jens Seeberg, "*Danske svin gør livet farligt for gravide og børn i Paraguay* [Danish pigs make life dangerous for pregnant women and children in Paraguay]," *Videnskab.dk,* February 6, 2019; Christian Erin-Madsen, "*Sojaens syge slagside* [The diseased lopsidedness of soy]," *DanWatch Report,* April 9,

2019; "*Produktion af soja til danske svin gør lokalbefolkningen alvorligt syg* [Production of soy for Danish pigs causes serious illness among the local population]," *Dr.dk*, April 13, 2019; "*Regnskov må lade livet for soja til danske grise* [Rainforests die to feed Danish pigs]," *Politiken*, April 23, 2019.

14. In connection to the use of antibiotics in food production, Denmark has lobbied for stricter EU regulations and reduced its own use of antibiotic growth promoters from 115,786 kilograms in 1994 to 12,283 in 1999 (Kirchhelle 2018, 8). In connection to eliminating deforestation, Denmark has been one of only five EU countries to work for the responsible management of agricultural supply chains and sustainable trade (Hansen et al. 2015).

15. See Weston (2018) for a vivid account of how humans experience and sense these ecological intimacies.

16. In the academic literature, these connections are powerfully demonstrated in Anna Tsing's 2015 study of a global supply chain of matsutake mushrooms and Donna Haraway's 2016 study of hormonal drugs.

17. This image of porous passages between body and environment has affinities with postindustrial theories of the metabolism as a regulatory zone that responds to environmental information and connects environments and organisms (Landecker 2011, 2013; Law and Mol 2008; Nicholson 2018; Solomon 2016; E. Wilson 2015). As Hannah Landecker notes, postindustrial theories of metabolism exist at a time in which "network," "communication," and "information" dominate the discursive realm (2013, 497–511). Theories of metabolism are not decoupled from historical time but are part of it. Within any given time, there has always been a traffic in conceptual resources between the biological and the social sciences.

18. In the 1950s, Denmark had 205,000 small farms. In 2017, less than 10,000 farms farmed the same land area and raised four times as many pigs (Kærgård 2017).

19. In an academic report, the labor market researchers Søren Andersen and Jonas Felbo-Kolding mentioned that the majority of Eastern European workers in Denmark worked in the country for a limited period and then returned to their home country (2013, 51). More recent news articles mention that an increased number of Eastern European workers—up to 50 percent—are still in the country after five years ("*Flere østeuropæere bosætter sig i Danmark* [More Eastern Europeans settle in Denmark]," *Dr.dk*, July 19, 2015; "*Nye tal: Antallet af østarbejdere slår alle rekorder* [New numbers: The number of Eastern European workers beats all records]," *Avisen.dk*, May 19, 2018; Henrik Jensen, "*Mange østeuropæere bliver boende i Danmark* [Many Eastern Europeans stay in Denmark]," *Berlingske Tidende*, July 18, 2015). The media have debated the pros and cons related to permanent residence and express the widespread expectation among Danes that foreign workers stay in Denmark only temporarily and return to their home countries.

20. Another study of intra-EU migration documents that EU migrants from Eastern Europe who take up work in Denmark occupy the lowest-paying occupations such as farming (Felbo-Kolding, Leschke, and Spreckelsen 2019).

21. According to EU legislation (European Union 2008), routine tail docking is illegal, yet tail docking may be practiced if pigs bite each other's tails. Tail biting is a behavior usually caused by a stressful environment that prevents pigs from using their foraging and investigative behavior, and it can be prevented by providing pigs with straw, hay, wood, mushrooms, or other kinds of enriching materials. In Denmark, 99 percent of the pigs reared per year in the country have their tails docked. In a number of EU countries, this action is systematically performed in the early days of the animal's life, despite the ban on routine tail docking.

22. Since 1993, there has been free movement of EU citizens within the EU member states. When EU citizens take up work in another member state, they have the right to equal treatment with national workers and thus gain access to welfare benefits such as those related to maternity or paternity, sickness, pension, studies, unemployment, becoming an invalid, and death (Remeur 2013). In Denmark since the beginning of the 2000s, concern about "welfare tourism" has been a subject of political debate, creating the public's belief that a large group of EU citizens are moving to Denmark to take advantage of the Danish welfare system and pose a great challenge to the Danish welfare state. A large quantitative study from 2018 refuted this belief, finding that nine out of ten EU citizens who receive welfare benefits in Denmark have lived in the country for two years or more and thus contributed to the public purse and had earned their way into the system at the time they received benefits (Martinsen, Rotger, Thierry 2019).

23. The minister was quoted in an article in the national Danish newspaper *Information*, which also reported that every third worker in the Danish farming industry came from abroad, mainly from Eastern Europe (Sille Veilmark, *"Dansk landbrug kan ikke hænge sammen uden østeuropæere* [Danish agriculture cannot function without Eastern Europeans]," *Information*, October 7, 2017).

24. Henrik Jensen, *"Tænketank: Vores velfærd kan ikke undvære østeuropæiske arbejdere* [Think tank: Our welfare cannot do without Eastern European workers]," *Berlingske Tidende*, December 15, 2019.

25. Denmark has a small population of 50–100 adult wild boars. In addition to building the fence, the government allowed hunters to shoot wild boars year-round.

26. Quoted in *"Vildsvinehegn ved grænsen får grønt lys* [Wild boar fence at the border has been approved]," *Berlingske Tidende*, June 4 2018. The amount of money mentioned by the minister referred to pig products exported to non-European countries.

27. The Danish People's Party was founded in 1995. It is characterized by being against immigration and skeptical about the European Union, and it supports the welfare state. In the 2001 election, the party won 12 percent of the votes. In the 2015 election, it won 21.1 percent of the votes, making it the party with the second-largest number of representatives in the parliament. In 2015 and 2016, the party played a decisive role in introducing temporary border controls at the Danish-German borders and implementing initiatives and regulations aimed at dissuading migrants from coming to Denmark. In the 2019 election, the party experienced a significant setback and won only 8.7 percent of the votes. The decline should not be interpreted as indicating a loss of public interest in the anti-immigration agenda in Danish politics. In fact, this agenda has been embraced by the Social Democratic Party and the center-right party, both mainstream parties.

28. Lærke Cramon *"Hegnet* [The fence]," *Information*, February 23, 2019; Erik Jensen, *"Danmark kom før Trump: Vi bygger hegn langs den tyske grænse for at beskytte os mod de vildsvin, ingen har set* [Denmark was ahead of Trump: We build a fence along the German border to protect ourselves from the wild boar which no one has seen]," *Politiken*, February 2, 2019.

29. When the bodies washed ashore, the fence was still being built, and thus there were passages for the boars to move across the German-Danish border on land.

30. Andrea Bisgaard, *"Endnu to døde vildsvin strandet på Ærø* [Two more dead wild boars have been stranded on Ærø]," *Fyns Amtsavis*, October 23, 2019; *"Døde vildsvin ved Ærø testes ikke for frygtet svinesygdom* [Dead wild boars are not being tested for dreaded swine disease]," *JydskeVestkysten*, October 24, 2019; Jakob Haislund, *"Døde vildsvin på Ærø har skabt debat om pesttest* [Dead wild boars on Ærø have raised debate on test for swine fever]," *Jyllands-Posten*, October 26, 2019; *"Ingen ved, hvorfor Ærø blev en vildsvineø* [No one knows why Ærø turned into a wild boar island]," *Fyns Amtsavis*, October 26, 2019; *"Ni døde vildsvin er skyllet op på Ærø* [Nine dead wild boars have washed ashore on the coasts of Ærø]," *Zetland*, October 29, 2019.

31. Quoted in Jakob Haislund, *"Døde vildsvin på Ærø har skabt debat om posttest."*

32. For example, in a 1970 publication titled "Equal Circumstances," one of Denmark's biggest workers' unions, *Dansk Arbejdsmand- og Specialarbejderforbund* [Danish Workers'

Union], said: "There is no foreign worker policy in the country. . . . It creates uncertainty and fear at the workplace where workers fear that the presence of foreign workers will lead to underpayment, pressure on social benefits, and risks of unemployment. At the same time, it becomes clear to everyone that foreign workers do not get the payment they as human beings have a right to" (*Der er ingen fremmedarbejderpolitik her i landet. . . . Det giver uro og ængstelse på arbejdspladsen, hvor man frygter, at tilstedeværelsen af for mange fremmedarbejdere medfører underbetaling, tryk på den sociale standard, og at tendens til arbejdsløshed bliver forstærket. For alle bliver det også mere klart, at fremmedarbejderne ikke får den behandling, de som mennesker kan gøre krav på*) (quoted in Jønsson 2018, 15).

33. The Immigration Act of 1983 provided the immigrant with the right to bring spouse, children under twenty, and parents to Denmark (Petersen and Jønsson 2013, 169). At the time it was considered one of the most liberal immigration laws in the world (Bissenbakker 2019).

34. Citizenship in Denmark is based on ethnic descent, which means that a newborn child has Danish citizenship if one or both parents do. For people who have not been born as Danish citizens, the path to citizenship is long. In 2021, the requirements were a minimum of nine years of continuous residence on Danish soil; documentation of active citizenship in Danish society; passing a citizenship exam; and having full-time work, proper housing conditions, no criminal record, fluency in Danish, and economic self-sufficiency (Danish Immigration Service, n.d.).

35. The quote is from the Danish Aliens Act of 2000 (law 208, paragraph 9, part 10). The attachment requirement was part of Danish immigration law until 2018. According to Mons Bissenbakker (2019), the requirement was tightened a number of times. For example, in 2002, the requirement, which had been that the couple's combined attachment to Denmark had to be at least equal to their attachment to any other country, changed. Now the couple's attachment to Denmark had to be greater than that to any other country. In 2016, the International Court of Human Rights ruled that the Danish way of using the attachment requirement was an act of indirect discrimination, which led to Denmark's abandoning the attachment requirement in 2018. However, in Danish immigration laws after 2018, the logics of national attachment continue to operate as the demands put on cohabitant and applicant have become increasingly strict (Bissenbakker 2019, 184).

36. Mikkel Rytter makes the argument that Danish immigration legislation is based on the "order of nature" (2010, 309) which David Schneider (1980) identified for Euro-American kinship. Danes who have a connection to the national community and the national territory through generations belong to the "order of nature," whereas immigrants belong to the "order of law" (Rytter 2010, 309), as their inclusion in the national community is based on purely juridical principles (eligibility for work permits, residence permits, or asylum), and legislation increasingly depicts them as people who do not belong because they do not share the Danes' history and cultural heritage.

37. Examples of regulation include cuts in social benefits to refugees and migrants by 45 percent (August 2015), the advertisement of benefit cuts in newspapers in Lebanon to discourage Lebanese from coming to Denmark (September 2015); and seizing of any assets exceeding $1,450 from asylum seekers to help pay for their subsistence in Denmark (January 2016).

38. For this short description of the effects of the deal with Turkey, I rely on reports from the British nongovernmental organization Choose Love (Long 2018) and Amnesty International (Amnesty International 2020). For discussions of how migrants' deaths and postmortem lives are extensions of political processes, see De Leon (2015).

39. In her ethnography of the border world in Ceuta, on the Moroccan coast, Perle Møhl (2020) describes a mutual surveillance on the part of migrants and border guards. The

migrants' border work involves scrutinizing fences and the routines and technologies of border guards, as well as coming to know the fences personally by being cut and snared by them when trying to climb over them. On the other side of the border, the guards' border work includes scrutinizing and surveillance using cameras and detection technologies that produce dots on screens in need of human interpretation. On both sides, border work is centered on reading signs.

40. As an example, in March 2019, responding to the situation of foreign fighters of Danish nationality returning to Denmark, Minister of Justice Søren Pape Poulsen said that Denmark was unable to deny them readmission but that "it would have been better if they had died in battle" (quoted in Emil Søndergård Ingvorsen, *"Pape om hjemvendte syrienskrigere: 'Det bedste ville være, at de var faldet i kamp'* [Pape on returned Syrian fighters: 'The best thing would be if the had fallen in battle']," *Dr. dk*, March 27, 2019.

41. In Danish, *"Med den såkaldte nødbremse kan vi midlertidigt lukke grænsen for asylansøgere, hvis der er tale om en krisesituation."* Quoted in Henrik Dannemand, *"Flygtningekrise: Regeringen er parat til at bruge 'asylnødbremsen'* [Refugee crisis: The government is ready to use the 'asylum brake']," *Berlingske Tidende*, March 1, 2020.

42. In Danish, *"Jeg tror ikke, at vi kan få et samfund til at fungere, hvis ikke alle, der bor her, er integrerede. Derfor bliver der nødt til at være en grænse for, hvor mange der kommer hertil"* (quoted in Jønsson 2018, 97).

43. In 2016, the Danish government adopted new rules that made people with temporary protection status wait for three years before applying for family reunification. In 2017, a report stated that it had been markedly difficult for disabled people to gain citizenship in Denmark. In 2014, 97 percent of applications were approved, but in 2017, the number had dropped to 4 percent. See Ulrik Dahlin, *"Det er blevet dramatisk sværere for handicappede at få dansk statsborgerskab* [It has become dramatically more difficult for disabled people to obtain Danish citizenship]," *Information*, October 31, 2017; Anton Geist, *"Danmark begår tilsyneladende konventionsbrud igen—og denne gang er det Folketinget, der står bag* [Denmark appears to be violating conventions again—and this time the Parliament is behind it]," *Information*, November 2, 2017.

44. In 2013, 91 percent of the children in Denmark one year old and 97 percent of children ages 3–5 attended publicly financed day care (Statistics Denmark 2014: https://ast.dk/filer /tal-og-undersogelser/tal-og-tendenser-filer/daginstitutioneri-de-nordiske-lande.pdf.)

45. In 2010, the Danish government launched an annual list of low-income enclaves named "ghettos" (*ghettoområder*), referring to neighborhoods in which more than half of the residents are from non-Western countries or descendants of migrants from non-Western countries, residents have a low educational level, residents have a weak connection to the labor market, and crime convictions are three times higher than the average. The 2018 Law on Education to Prevent Parallel Societies was part of a cluster of laws to enhance integration in areas that legislators refer to as "ghettos" and "deprived enclaves" (*udsatte boligområder*).

46. In Danish, *Aftale mellem regeringen (Venstre, Liberal Alliance og Konservative), Socialdemokratiet og Dansk Folkeparti om delaftale på Børne- og Socialministeriets område om obligatorisk læringstilbud til 1-årige i udsatte boligområder og skærpet straf for pligtforsømmelse for ledere i offentlig tjeneste eller hverv.*

47. The notion of the body politic goes back to medieval times, when the king's body was seen as both a biological organism and an embodiment of the political community (Kermode 2000). In the nineteenth and early twentieth centuries, the image of society as organism loomed large in the theories of Karl Marx and Talcott Parsons, for example.

48. Bermant (2017) makes a similar argument in her study of border politics and practices in the Spanish enclave of Melilla, in northeastern Morocco. She argues that mobility and

immobility do not represent opposing interests but are two sides of the same system that serves global capitalism.

49. In a national survey covering the period 2011–2013, the average annual intake of meat among Danes ages 4–75 was fifty-two kilos. Pork constituted 66 percent of that amount (Fagt, Matthiessen, and Biltoft-Jensen 2018).

50. In 2009, the Danish People's Party branch in a municipality close to Copenhagen suggested that a minimum of 20 percent of the meals served in public institutions had to contain Danish pork (Mikkel Bahl, "*DF'er: Hver femte ret skal være med svin* [DF'er: One in five meals should contain pork]," *Politiken*, November 6, 2009).

51. Quoted in Jesper Vangkilde, "*Thorning går ind i frikadellekrigen* [Thorning enters the meatball war]," *Politiken*, August 11, 2013.

52. Quoted in "'*Frikadellekrigen' i Randers er afgjort: Krav om svinekød på institutioner* ['The Meat Ball War' in Randers is settled: Demand for pork in institutions]," *Jyllandsposten*, January 18, 2016. In addition to that quote from a national newspaper, a local newspaper quoted Frank Nørgaard, a council member, as saying, "We will ensure that Danish children and youth can have pork in the future" (Karin Hede Pedersen, "*Nu skal der serveres gris i de kommunale institutioner* [From now on pork will be served in municipal institutions]," *Randers Amtsavis*, January 18, 2016).

53. Quoted in "*DF vil tvinge skoler til at servere svinekød* [DF wants to force schools to serve pork]," *Altinget*, May 29, 2018.

54. Sarah Ives's fascinating *Steeped in Heritage* (2017) describes similar processes in South Africa in relation to rooibos tea.

55. Quoted in Jens Ejsing, "*S: Flæskeforbud skader integrationen i København* [Social Democrats: Ban on pork hinders integration in Copenhagen]," *Berlingske Tidende*, February 11, 2015.

56. "*Velfærd kan blive det nye bacon* [Welfare may become the new bacon]," *Berlingske Tidende*, January 8, 2014.

REFERENCES

Agamben, Giorgio. 1998. *Homo Sacer: Sovereign Power and Bare Life*. Translated by Daniel Heller-Roazen. Stanford, CA: Stanford University Press.

Ahmed, Sara. 2019. *What's the Use? On the Uses of Use*. Durham, NC: Duke University Press.

Amnesty International. 2020. "Trapped in the EU's New Refugee Camp: Greece." Amnesty International, January 27. https://www.amnesty.org.uk/trapped-europe-new-refugee-camp -greece.

Andersen, Anders D., Per T. Sangild, Sara L. Munch, Eline M. van der Beek, Ingrid B. Renes, Chris van Ginneken et al. 2016. "Delayed Growth, Motor Function and Learning in Preterm Pigs during Early Postnatal Life." *American Journal Regul Integr Comp Physiol* 310: R481–492.

Andersen, Jørgen Goul. 2019. "Denmark: The Welfare State as a Victim of Neoliberal Economic Failure?" In *Welfare and the Great Recession: A Comparative Study*, edited by Stefán Ólafsson, Mary Daly, Olli Kangas, and Joakim Palme, 192–209. Oxford: Oxford University Press.

Andersen, Søren Kaj, and Jonas Felbo-Kolding. 2013. *Danske virksomheders brug af østeuropæisk arbejdskraft* [The Use of Eastern European Labor by Danish Companies]. Copenhagen: Employment Relations Research Centre (FAOS).

Anderson, Benedict. 2006. *Imagined Communities: Reflections on the Origin and Spread of Nationalism*. London: Verso Books.

Ankeny, Rachel A., and Sabina Leonelli. 2016. "Repertoires: A Post-Kuhnian Perspective on Scientific Change and Collaborative Research." *Studies in History and Philosophy of Science Part A*, 60 (December): 18–28.

Anneberg, Inger, and Nils Bubandt. 2016. "Dyrevelfærdsstaten: Grisens krop, velfærdens historie og selve livets politik i Danmark [The Animal Welfare State: The Pig's Body, the History of Welfare and the Politics of Life Itself in Denmark]." *Tidsskriftet Antropologi* 73: 111–136.

Anneberg, Inger, and Mette Vaarst. 2018. "Farm Animals in a Welfare State: Commercial Pigs in Denmark." In *Domestication Gone Wild: Politics and Practices of Multispecies Relations*, edited by Heather A. Swanson, Marianne E. Lien, and Gro B. Ween, 94–116. Durham, NC: Duke University Press.

Anneberg, Inger, Mette Vaarst, and Nils Bubandt. 2013. "Pigs and Profits: Hybrids of Animals, Technology and Humans in Danish Industrialised Farming." *Social Anthropology* 21 (4): 542–559.

Asad, Talal. 2000. "Agency and Pain: An Exploration." *Culture and Religion* 1 (1): 29–60.

Barndt, Deborah. 2008. *Tangled Routes: Women, Work, and Globalization on the Tomato Trail*. Plymouth, UK: Rowman and Littlefield.

Barrett, Barbara Ann. 2016. "Guidelines in Action in Prenatal Screening. A Study of Organisational Standardisation and Clinical Management of Risk Markers in Routine First Trimester Screening in Denmark." PhD diss., University of Copenhagen.

Bendixen, Emøke, Marianne Danielsen, Knud Larsen, and Christian Bendixen. 2010. "Advances in Porcine Genomics and Proteomics—A Toolbox for Developing the Pig as a Model Organism for Molecular Biomedical Research." *Briefings in Functional Genomics* 9 (3): 208–219.

Bendixsen, Synnove, Mary Bente Bringslid, and Halvard Vike. 2018. "Introduction: Egalitarianism in a Scandinavian Context." In *Egalitarianism in Scandinavia: Historical and Contemporary Perspectives*, edited by Synnove Bendixsen, Mary Bente Bringslid, and Halvard Vike, 1–44. Cham, Switzerland: Palgrave Macmillan.

Bermant, Laia Soto. 2017. "The Mediterranean Question: Europe and Its Predicament in the Southern Peripheries." In *The Borders of "Europe": Autonomy of Migration, Tactics of Bordering*, edited by Nicholas De Genova, 120–140. Durham, NC: Duke University Press.

Bharadwaj, Aditya. 2008. "Biosociality and Biocrossings: Encounters with Assisted Conception and Embryonic Cells in India." In *Biosocialities, Genetics and the Social Sciences: Making Biologies and Identities*, edited by Sahra Gibbon and Carlos Novas, 98–116. London: Routledge.

Birke, Linda. 2003. "Who—or What—Are the Rats (and Mice) in the Laboratory?" *Society and Animals* 11 (3): 207–224.

Bissenbakker, Mons. 2019. "Attachment Required: The Affective Governmentality of Marriage Migration in the Danish Aliens Act 2000–2018." *International Political Sociology* 13 (2): 181–197.

Blanchette, Alex. 2020. *Porkopolis: American Animality, Standardized Life, and the Factory Farm*. Durham, NC: Duke University Press.

Bloch, Maurice. 1992. *Prey into Hunter: The Politics of Religious Experience*. Cambridge: Cambridge University Press.

Block, Laura. 2015. "Regulating Membership: Explaining Restriction and Stratification of Family Migration in Europe." *Journal of Family Issues* 36 (11): 1433–1452.

Bollen, Peter J. A., Axel K. Hansen, and Aage K. O. Alstrup. 2010. *The Laboratory Swine*. Boca Raton, FL: CRC Press.

Borring, Julie, and Ditte S. Hansen. 2017. "Milk Sharing and Exchange Relations." MA thesis, University of Copenhagen.

Borring, Julie, Ditte S. Hansen, Mie S. Dam, and Mette N. Svendsen. 2018. "Fra modermælk til donormælk: Forhandlinger af mælk, individ og velfærdskollektiv [From Mother's Milk to Donor Milk: Negotiations of Milk, Individual, and Welfare Collective]." *Tidsskrift for Forskning i Sygdom og Samfund* 15 (29): 99–119.

Brosnan, Caragh, and Mike Michael. 2014. "Enacting the Neuro in Practice: Translational Research, Adhesion and the Promise of Porosity." *Social Studies of Science* 44 (5): 680–700.

Bruns, Gerald L. 2011. *On Ceasing to Be Human*. Stanford, CA: Stanford University Press.

Buller, Henry. 2014. "Animal Geographies I." *Progress in Human Geography* 38 (2): 308–318.

Butler, Judith. 2006. *Precarious Life: The Powers of Mourning and Violence*. London: Verso Books.

———. 2016. *Frames of War: When Is Life Grievable?* London: Verso Books.

Caliebe, Amke, Almut Nebel, Cheryl Makarewicz, Michael Krawczak, and Ben Krause-Kyora. 2017. "Insights into Early Pig Domestication Provided by Ancient DNA Analysis." *Scientific Reports* 7 (44550): 1–6.

Candea, Matei. 2010. "'I Fell in Love with Carlos the Meerkat': Engagement and Detachment in Human-Animal Relations." *American Ethnologist* 37 (2): 241–258.

Capital Region [Region Hovedstaden]. N.d. "Modtagelse af immature og premature børn med GA 23 + 0 − 33 + 6, indledende behandling [Admission of Immature and Premature Infants with GA 23 + 0 − 33 + 6, Initial Treatment]." Accessed April 23, 2021. https://vip.regionh.dk/VIP/Admin/GUI.nsf/Desktop.html?open&openlink=http://vip.regionh.dk/VIP/Slutbruger/Portal.nsf/Main.html?open&unid=X81CB8E291B283DD1C1257915 0077ECE5&dbpath=/VIP/Redaktoer/130147.nsf/&windowwidth=1100&windowheight=600&windowtitle=S%F8gTry.

Carroll, Katherine E. 2016. "The Milk of Human Kinship: Donated Breast Milk in Neonatal Intensive Care." In *Critical Kinship Studies: Kinship (Trans)Formed*, edited by Charlotte Kr"løkke, Lene Myong, Stine W. Adrian, and Tine Tjørnhøj-Thomsen, 15–31. London: Rowman and Littlefield.

Carsten, Janet. 1995. "The Substance of Kinship and the Heat of the Hearth: Feeding, Personhood, and Relatedness among Malays in Pulau Langkawi." *American Ethnologist* 22 (2): 223–241.

———. 1997. *The Heat of the Hearth: The Process of Kinship in a Malay Fishing Community.* Oxford: Oxford University Press.

Changing Markets Foundation. 2018. *Growing the Good: The Case for Low-Carbon Transition in the Food Sector.* Utrecht, the Netherlands: Changing Markets Foundation.

Christiansen, Niels Finn, and Klaus Petersen. 2001. "The Dynamics of Social Solidarity: The Danish Welfare State, 1900–2000." *Scandinavian Journal of History* 26 (3): 177–196.

Christoffersen-Deb, Astrid. 2012. "Viability: A Cultural Calculus of Personhood at the Beginnings of Life." *Medical Anthropology Quarterly* 26 (4): 575–594.

Chrulew, Matthew. 2013. "Preventing and Giving Death at the Zoo: Heini Hediger's 'Death Due to Behaviour.'" In *Animal Death*, edited by Jay Johnston and Fiona Probyn-Rapsey, 221–238. Sydney, Australia: Sydney University Press.

Clark, Nigel. 2007. "Animal Interface: The Generosity of Domestication." In *Where the Wild Things Are Now: Domestication Reconsidered*, edited by Rebecca Cassidy and Molly Mullin, 49–70. Oxford: Berg.

Clarke, Adele. 1998. *Disciplining Reproduction: Modernity, American Life Sciences, and the Problems of Sex.* Berkeley: University of California Press.

Cooper, Melinda, and Catherine Waldby. 2014. *Clinical Labor: Tissue Donors and Research Subjects in the Global Bioeconomy.* Durham, NC: Duke University Press.

Coopmans, Catelijne, and Karen M. McNamara. 2020. "Care in Translation: Care-ful Research in Medical Settings." *East Asian Science, Technology, and Society* 14 (1): 1–14.

Copenhagen University Hospital. 2015 "Familien [The Family]." https://www.rigshospitalet .dk/afdelinger-og-klinikker/julianemarie/videnscenter-for-tidligt-foedte-boern/neonat alafdelingen/Sider/Familien.aspx.

———. N.d. . "Mælkevejen [The Milky Way]." https://www.rigshospitalet.dk/afdelinger-og -klinikker/julianemarie/videnscenter-for-amning-af-boern/viden/Sider/maelkevejen .aspx.

Dalgaard, Lars. 2014. "Comparison of Minipig, Dog, Monkey and Human Drug Metabolism and Disposition." *Journal of Pharmacological and Toxicological Methods* 74 (July-August): 80–92.

Dam, Mie S., Sandra M. Juhl, Per T. Sangild, and Mette N. Svendsen. 2017. "Feeding Premature Neonates: Kinship and Species in Translational Neonatology." *Social Science and Medicine* 179 (April): 129–136.

Dam, Mie S., Per T. Sangild, and Mette N. Svendsen. 2018. "Translational Neonatology Research: Transformative Encounters across Species and Disciplines." *History and Philosophy of the Life Sciences* 40 (21): 1–16.

———. 2020. "Plastic Pigs and Public Secrets in Translational Neonatology in Denmark." *Palgrave Communications* 6 (84): 1–10.

Dam, Mie S., and Mette N. Svendsen. 2018. "Treating Piglets: Balancing Standardization and Individual Treatments in Translational Neonatology Research." *BioSocieties* 13 (2): 349–367.

DanBred, 2018. "DanBred Breeding Goals and Documented Results." https://danbred.com /en/danbred-breeding-goals-and-documented-results.

Danish Agriculture and Food Council. N.d. "The Danish Agriculture and Food Council." Accessed March 19, 2021. https://agricultureandfood.dk/about-us/focus.

———. July 2019. "Statistics 2018 Pigmeat." Accessed April 14, 2021. https://lf.dk/-/media/lf/tal-og-analyser/aarsstatistikker/statistik-svin/2018/2018-a5-statistik-svin-en-v2.pdf.

———. June 2020. "Statistics 2019 Pigmeat." Accessed April 9, 2021. https://lf.dk/-/media/lf/tal-og-analyser/aarsstatistikker/statistik-svin/2019/ny-version/2020-a5-statistik-gris-en-digital-final.pdf.

Danish Government. 2016. "A Stronger Denmark: Controlling the Influx of Refugees." https://uim.dk/filer/nyheder-2016/a-stronger-danmark-in-english.pdf.

Danish Health Authority. 2004. "Retningslinjer for fosterdiagnostik - prænatal information, risikovurdering, rådgivning og diagnostik [Guidelines for Prenatal Diagnostics—Prenatal Information, Risk Assessment, Counselling and Diagnostics]."

———. 2009. "Anbefalinger for svangreomsorgen 2009" [Guidelines for Pregnancy Care 2009]." https://docplayer.dk/2245703-Anbefalinger-for-svangreomsorgen.html.

———. 2012. "Vejledning om forudgående fravalg af livsforlængende behandling, herunder genoplivningsforsøg, og om afbrydelse af behandling [Guidelines Concerning Refusal of Life-Extending Treatment, including Resuscitation Attempts, and Ceasing of Treatment]." Copenhagen: Danish Patient Safety Authority.

———. 2013. "Anbefalinger for Svangreomsorgen 2013 [Guidelines for Pregnancy Care 2013]." https://www.sst.dk/-/media/Udgivelser/2015/Anbefalinger-svangreomsorgen/Anbefalinger-for-svangreomsorgen.ashx?la=da&hash=757F1953C4B437A70A44024B32D7DD2E1B0A9F5B.

———. 2017. "Retningslinjer for fosterdiagnostik [Guidelines for Prenatal Diagnosis]." Copenhagen: Danish Board of Health.

Danish Health Data Authority [Sundhedsdatastyrelsen]. 2021. *Assisteret reproduktion 2019* [Assisted Reproduction 2019]. Copenhagen: The Danish Health Data Authority.

Danish Immigration Service. N.d. "Danish citizenship." Accessed April 27, 2021. https://nyidanmark.dk/en-GB/Words%20and%20Concepts%20Front%20Page/Shared/Danish%20citizenship.

Danish Ministry of External Affairs. 1978. "Bekendtgørelse af konvention af 22. januar 1976 med Tyrkiet om social sikring [Government Order with Turkey about Social Security]." https://www.retsinformation.dk/Forms/R0710.aspx?id=84236.

———. 1979. "Bekendtgørelse af konvention af 22. juni 1977 med Jugoslavien om social sikring [Government Order with Yugoslavia about Social Security]." https://www.retsinformation.dk/Forms/R0710.aspx?id=53510.

Danish Ministry of Food, Agriculture and Fisheries. 2012. *Avl af Svin* [Breeding of Pigs]. Delrapport afgivet af arbejdsgruppen om avl af dyr [Progress Report by Working Group on Animal Breeding]. Copenhagen: Danish Ministry of Food, Agriculture and Fisheries.

Danish Ministry of Higher Education and Science. 2018. "About the Council." Accessed April 14, 2021. https://ufm.dk/en/research-and-innovation/councils-and-commissions/former-councils-and-commissions/the-danish-council-for-strategic-research/about-the-council.

Danish Ministry of Interior Affairs. 1977. "Betænkning om prænatal genetisk diagnostik [White Paper on Prenatal Genetic Diagnostics]." Copenhagen: Statens Trykningskontor.

———. 1984. *Fremskridtets pris* [The Price of Progress]. Copenhagen: Ministry of Interior Affairs.

Danish Ministry of Taxation. 2018. "Skatteøkonomisk Redegørelse [Tax Financial Statement]." Copenhagen: Ministry of Taxation.

Davies, Gail. 2012. "What Is a Humanized Mouse? Remaking the Species and Spaces of Translational Medicine." *Body and Society* 18 (3–4): 126–155.

Davies, Gail, Beth Greenhough, Pru Hobson-West, and Robert G. W. Kirk. 2018. "Science, Culture, and Care in Laboratory Animal Research: Interdisciplinary Perspectives on the History and Future of the 3Rs." *Science, Technology, and Human Values* 43 (4): 603–621.

De Genova, Nicholas. 2017. "Introduction: The Borders of 'Europe' and the European Question." In *The Borders of "Europe": Autonomy of Migration, Tactics of Bordering*, edited by Nicholas De Genova, 1–35. Durham, NC: Duke University Press.

De Leon, Jason. 2015. *The Land of Open Graves: Living and Dying on the Migrant Trail*. Oakland: University of California Press.

De Sousa, Ivan Sergio Freire, and Rita de Cássia Milagres Teixeira Vieira. 2008. "Soybeans and Soyfoods in Brazil, with Notes on Argentina: Sketch of an Expanding World Commodity." In *The World of Soy*, edited by Christine M. Du Bois, Chee-Beng Tan, and Sidney Mintz, 234–256. Urbana: University of Illinois Press.

Derrida, Jacques. 2008. *The Gift of Death and Literature in Secret*. Translated by David Wills. Chicago: University of Chicago Press.

Despret, Vinciane. 2008. "The Becomings of Subjectivity in Animal Worlds." *Subjectivity* 23 (1): 123–139.

———. 2016. *What Would Animals Say If We Asked the Right Questions?* Minneapolis: University of Minnesota Press.

Druglitrø, Tone. 2016. "Care and Tinkering in the Animal House: Conditioning Monkeys for Poliomyelitis Research and Public Health Work." In *Animal Housing and Human-Animal Relations: Politics, Practices and Infrastructures*, edited by Kristian Bjørkdahl and Tone Druglitrø, 151–166. London: Routledge.

———. 2018. "'Skilled Care' and the Making of Good Science." *Science, Technology, and Human Values* 43 (4): 649–670.

Durkheim, Emile. 1915. *The Elementary Forms of the Religious Life*. Translated by Joseph Ward Swain. Oxford: Oxford University Press.

Dyrenes Beskyttelse. "Fakta om avl for større kuld og pattegrisedødlighed [Facts about Breeding for Larger Litters and Piglet Mortality]." June 2, 2010.

Edwards, A. David, Peter Brocklehurst, Alistair J. Gunn, Henry Halliday, Edmund Juszczak, Malcom Levene, Brenda Strohm, et al. 2010. "Neurological Outcomes at 18 Months of Age after Moderate Hypothermia for Perinatal Hypoxic Ischaemic Encephalopathy: Synthesis and Meta-Analysis of Trial Data." *BMJ* 340: c363.

Edwards, Jeanette, Sarah Franklin, Eric Hirsch, and Frances Price. 1999. *Technologies of Procreation: Kinship in the Age of Assisted Conception*. London: Routledge.

Einhorn, Eric S., and John Logue. 2003. *Modern Welfare States: Scandinavian Politics and Policy in the Global Age*. Westport, CT: Praeger.

Eskildsen, Maria, and Andreas V. Weber. 2018. *Svineproduktion* [Pig Production]. 3rd ed. Aarhus, Denmark: SEGES Forlag.

European Union. 2008. "Council Directive 2008/120/EC, 18 December on Laying Down Minimum Standards for the Protection of Pigs." Accessed April 28, 2021. https://eur-lex.europa.eu/legal-content/EN/TXT/PDF/?uri=CELEX:32008L0120&from=HR.

———. 2010. "Directive 2010/63/EU of the European Parliament and of the Council of 22 September 2010 on the Protection of Animals Used for Scientific Purposes." Accessed April 27 2021. https://ec.europa.eu/environment/chemicals/lab_animals/legislation_en.htm.

Fagt, Sisse, Jeppe Matthiessen, and Anja Pia Biltoft-Jensen. 2018. "Hvor meget kød spiser danskerne?—data fra statistikker og kostundersøgelser [How Much Meat Do the Danes Eat?—Data from Statistics and Dietary Studies]." *DTU Fødevareinstitutet* 2018 (4): 1–6. https://backend.orbit.dtu.dk/ws/portalfiles/portal/162456892/E_artikel_Hvor_meget_koed_spiser_danskerne.pdf.

Fassin, Didier. 2018. *Life: A Critical User's Manual*. Cambridge: Policy Press.

Felbo-Kolding, Jonas, Janine Leschke, and Thees F. Spreckelsen. 2019. "A Division of Labour? Labour Market Segmentation by Region of Origin: The Case of Intra-EU Migrants in the UK, Germany and Denmark." *Journal of Ethnic and Migration Studies* 45 (15): 2820–2843.

Felt, Ulrike, Milena D. Bister, Michael Strassing, and Ursula Wagner. 2009. "Refusing the Information Paradigm: Informed Consent, Medical Research, and Patient Participation." *Health* 13 (1): 87–106.

Ferry, Elizabeth Emma, and Mandana E. Limbert. 2008. Introduction to *Timely Assets: The Politics of Resources and Their Temporalities*, edited by Elizabeth Emma Ferry and Mandana E. Limbert, 3–24. Santa Fe, NM: School for Advanced Research Press.

Fischer, Bob. 2020. Introduction to *The Routledge Handbook of Animal Ethics*, edited by Bob Fischer, 1–17. New York: Routledge.

Fong, Vanessa L. 2004. *Only Hope: Coming of Age under China's One-Child Policy*. Stanford, CA: Stanford University Press.

Foucault, Michel. 1990 [1976]. *The History of Sexuality Volume 1: An Introduction*. Translated by Robert Hurley. New York: Vintage Books.

Frank, Arthur W. 2010. *Letting Stories Breathe: A Socio-Narratology*. Chicago: University of Chicago Press.

Franklin, Sarah. 1997. *Embodied Progress: A Cultural Account of Assisted Conception*. London: Routledge.

———. 2007. *Dolly Mixtures: The Remaking of Genealogy*. Durham, NC: Duke University Press.

———. 2012. "Anthropology of Biomedicine and Bioscience." In *The SAGE Handbook of Social Anthropology*, edited by Richard Fardon, Olivia Harris, Trevor H. J. Marchand, Mark Nuttall, Cris Shore, Veronica Strang, Richard A. Wilson, 42–55. London: SAGE Publications.

Franklin, Sarah, and Celia Roberts. 2006. *Born and Made: An Ethnography of Preimplantation Genetic Diagnosis*. Princeton, NJ: Princeton University Press.

Frederiksen, Mette. 2020a. "Pressemøde den 11. marts 2020 [Press Conference on 11 March 2020]." Accessed April 27, 2021. https://www.stm.dk/statsministeren/taler/statsminister-mette-frederiksens-indledning-paa-pressemoede-i-statsministeriet-om-corona-virus-den-11-marts-2020/.

———. 2020b. "Pressemøde den 15. marts 2020 [Press Conference on 15 March 2020]." Accessed April 27, 2021. https://www.stm.dk/presse/pressemoedearkiv/pressemoede-den-15-marts-2020/.

Freud, Sigmund. 1978 [1919]. "The Uncanny." In *The Standard Edition of the Complete Psychological Works of Sigmund Freud*. Vol. 7: *An Infantile Neurosis and Other Works*. Translated and edited by James Strachey, Anna Freud, Alix Strachey, and Alan Tyson, 217–252. London: Hogarth.

Friese, Carrie. 2013a. *Cloning Wild Life: Zoos, Captivity, and the Future of Endangered Animals*. New York: New York University Press.

———. 2013b. "Realizing Potential in Translational Medicine: The Uncanny Emergence of Care as Science." *Current Anthropology* 54 (S7): S129–S138.

———. 2019. "Intimate Entanglements in the Animal House: Caring for and about Mice." *Sociological Review* 67 (2): 287–298.

Friese, Carrie, and Adele Clarke. 2012. "Transposing Bodies of Knowledge and Technique: Animal Models at Work in Reproductive Sciences." *Social Studies of Science* 42 (1): 31–52.

Friese, Carrie, and Joanna Latimer. 2019. "Entanglements in Health and Well-Being: Working with Model Organisms in Biomedicine and Bioscience." *Medical Anthropology Quarterly* 33 (1): 120–137.

Fritzbøger, Bo. 2015. *Mellem land og by: Landbohøjskolens historie* [Between Country and City: the History of the Agricultural School]. Copenhagen: Science Communication.

Gammeltoft, Tine M. 2014. *Haunting Images: A Cultural Account of Selective Reproduction in Vietnam*. Berkeley: University of California Press.

Gammeltoft, Tine M., and Ayo Wahlberg. 2014. "Selective Reproductive Technologies." *Annual Review of Anthropology* 43: 201–216.

Geissler, Paul W. 2013. "Public Secrets in Public Health: Knowing Not to Know while Making Scientific Knowledge." *American Ethnologist* 40 (1): 13–34.

Girard, René. 1977. *Violence and the Sacred*. Translated by Patrick Gregory. Baltimore, MD: Johns Hopkins University Press.

Gjerløff, Anne Kathrine, and Tenna V. Jensen. 2010. "Svin—kvalitet og kontrol [Pig—Quality and Control]." *Akademisk kvarter|Academic Quarter* 1: 52–60.

Gjødsbøl, Iben M., Lene Koch, and Mette N. Svendsen. 2017. "Resisting Decay: On Disposal, Valuation, and Care in a Dementia Nursing Home in Denmark." *Social Science and Medicine* 184 (July): 116–123.

Govindrajan, Radhika. 2015. "'The Goat That Died for Family': Animal Sacrifice and Interspecies Kinship in India's Central Himalayas." *American Ethnologist* 42 (3): 504–519.

———. 2018. *Animal Intimacies: Interspecies Relatedness in India's Central Himalayas*. Chicago: University of Chicago Press.

Greisen, Gorm, and Tine B. Henriksen. 2018. "Don't Rush It: Conservative Care in Denmark." *Pediatrics* 142 (supplement 1): S539–S544.

Griffin, Roger. 2007. *Modernism and Fascism: The Sense of a Beginning under Mussolini and Hitler*. New York: Palgrave Macmillan.

Groenen, Martien A. M., Alan L. Archibald, Hirohide Uenishi, Christopher K. Tuggle, Yasuhiro Takeuchi, Max F. Rothschild, Claire Rogel-Gaillard, et al. 2012. "Analyses of the Pig Genomes Provide Insight into Porcine Demography and Evolution." *Nature* 491: 393–398.

Gullestad, Marianne. 2002. "Invisible Fences: Egalitarianism, Nationalism and Racism." *Royal Anthropological Institute* 8 (1): 45–63.

Gutierrez, Karina, Naomi Dicks, Werner G. Glanzner, Luis B. Agellon, and Vilceu Bordignon. 2015. "Efficacy of the Porcine Species in Biomedical Research." *Frontiers in Genetics* 6 (293): 1–9.

Hamann, Karen. 2006. "An Overview of Danish Pork Industry: Integration and Structure." *Advances in Pork Production* 17: 93–97.

Hansen, Eva Kjer, Ségolène Royal, Gerd Müller, Lillian Ploumen, Vidar Helgesen, and Justine Greening. "Amsterdam Declaration, Towards Eliminating Deforestation from Agricultural Commodity Chains with European Countries." December 7, 2015. European Union. Accessed April 20, 2021. https://www.proterrafoundation.org/wp-content/uploads/2017/07/AmsterdamDeclarationDeforestation26Agro-commoditychains.pdf.

Hansen, Lene. 2002. "Sustaining Sovereignty: The Danish Approach to Europe." In *European Integration and National Identity: The Challenge of the Nordic States*, edited by Lene Hansen and Ole Waever, 50–87. London: Routledge.

Haraway, Donna J. 1989. *Primate Visions: Gender, Race and Nature in the World of Modern Science*. London: Routledge.

———. 1997. *Modest_Witness@Second_Millenium: FemaleMan_Meets_ OncoMouse: Feminism and Technoscience*. New York: Routledge.

———. 2003. *The Companion Species Manifesto: Dogs, People, and Significant Otherness*. Chicago: Prickly Paradigm Press.

———. 2008. *When Species Meet*. Minneapolis: University of Minnesota Press.

————. 2016. *Staying with the Trouble: Making Kin in the Chthulucene*. Durham, NC: Duke University Press.

Harrison, Ruth. 1964. *Animal Machines: The New Factory Farming Industry*. London: Vincent Stuart.

Haugegaard, John. 2006. "Avlens indflydelse på danske svins velfærd [The Influence of Breeding on the Welfare of Danish Pigs]." *Dansk Veterinærtidsskrift* 89 (8): 10–13.

Heinsen, Laura L. 2018. "Moral Adherers: Pregnant Women Undergoing Routine Prenatal Screening in Denmark." In *Selective Reproduction in the 21st Century*, edited by Ayo Wahlberg and Tine M. Gammeltoft, 69–95. Cham, Switzerland: Palgrave Macmillan.

Helmreich, Stefan. 2009. *Alien Ocean: Anthropological Voyages in Microbial Seas*. Berkeley: University of California Press.

Henriksen, Ingrid, and Niels Kærgård. 2014. "Dansk landbrugs største og mest succesfulde omstilling [The Largest and Most Successful Conversion of Danish Agriculture]." *Tidsskrift for Landøkonomi* 200 (2): 169–178.

Hetherington, Kevin. 2004. "Secondhandedness: Consumption, Disposal, and Absent Presence." *Environment and Planning D* 22 (1): 157–173.

Hetherington, Kregg. 2013. "Beans before the Law: Knowledge Practices, Responsibility, and the Paraguayan Soy Boom." *Cultural Anthropology* 28 (1): 65–85.

————. 2020. *The Government of Beans: Regulating Life in the Age of Monocrops*. Durham, NC: Duke University Press.

Hinchliffe, Stephen, Mark Jackson, Katrina Wyatt, Anne E. Barlow, Manuela Barreto, Linda Clare, Michael H. Depledge, et al. 2018. "Healthy Publics: Enabling Cultures and Environments for Health." *Humanities and Social Science Communications* 4 (57): 1–10.

Hinterberger, Amy. 2018. "Marked 'H' for Human: Chimeric Life and the Politics of the Human." *BioSocieties* 13 (2): 453–469.

Hird, Myra J. 2004. "Chimerism, Mosaicism and the Cultural Construction of Kinship." *Sexualities* 7 (2): 217–232.

Hoeyer, Klaus. 2005. "The Role of Ethics in Commercial Genetic Research: Notes on the Notion of Commodification." *Medical Anthropology* 24 (1): 45–70.

————. 2013. *Exchanging Human Bodily Material: Rethinking Bodies and Markets*. Dordrecht: Springer.

————. 2017. Suspense. Reflections on the Cryopolitics of the Body. In *Cryopolitics. Frozen Life in a Melting World*, edited by Joanna Radin and Emma Kowal, 205–214. Cambridge, MA: MIT Press

Hogle, L. 2022. "Enacting Authenticity: Changing Ontologies of Biological Entities." In *The Palgrave Handbook of the Anthropology of Technology*, edited by Maja Hojer Bruun, Ayo Wahlberg, Rachel Douglas-Jones, Cathrine Hasse, Klaus Hoeyer, Dorthe Brogård Kristensen, and Brit Ross Winthereik. Singapore: Palgrave Macmillan

Holmberg, Tora. 2008. "A Feeling for the Animal: On Becoming an Experimentalist." *Society and Animals* 16 (4): 316–335.

Holmstrup, Gitte, Johannes Schjelde, Rikke Lundsgaard, Thyge Nygaard, Lisbet Ogstrup, and Birgitte Iversen Damm. 2018. *Sådan ligger landet—Tal om landbrug 2017* [This Is How the Country Is—Numbers on Agriculture 2017]. Copenhagen: Dyrenes Beskyttelse.

Hubert, Henri, and Marcel Mauss. 1968. *Sacrifice: Its Nature and Functions*. Translated by W. D. Halls. London: Cohen and West.

Hviid, Kirsten. 2010. "'Like Winning a Prize in the Lottery': Social Strategies amongst Irregular Ukrainian Trainees Working in the Danish Agricultural Sector." In *Irregular Migration in a Scandinavian Perspective*, edited by Martin Bak Jørgensen, Trine Lund Thomsen, Susi Meret, Kirsten Hviid, and Helle Stenum, 179–203. Maastricht, the Netherlands: Shaker.

Høyer, Morten. 2018. Letter from Danish Agriculture and Food Council to the Environment and Food Committee in the Danish Parliament, July 27, 2018.

Ikegami, Machiko, Alan Jobe, and Theodore Glatz. 1981. "Surface Activity Following Surfactant Treatment in Premature Lambs." *Journal of Applied Physiology* 51 (2): 306–312.

Innovation Fund Denmark. N.d. "Innovation Fund Denmark's Politically Determined Focus Areas." Accessed 19 April 2021. https://innovationsfonden.dk/en/news-press-jobs/inno vation-fund-denmarks-politically-determined-focus-areas.

Ives, Sarah F. 2017. *Steeped in Heritage: The Racial Politics of South African Rooibos Tea.* Durham, NC: Duke University Press.

Jackson, Michael. 1998. *Minima Ethnographica: Intersubjectivity and the Anthropological Project.* Chicago: Chicago University Press.

Jain, S. Lochlann. 2010. "The Mortality Effect: Counting the Dead in the Cancer Trial." *Public Culture* 22 (1): 89–117.

Jenkins, Richard. 2011. *Being Danish: Paradoxes of Identity in Everyday Life.* Copenhagen: Museum Tusculanum Press.

Jensen, Anja Marie Bornø. 2016. "'Make Sure Somebody Will Survive from This': Transformative Practices of Hope among Danish Organ Donor Families." *Medical Anthropology Quarterly* 30(3): 378–394.

Jensen, Anja Marie Bornø, and Mette N. Svendsen. 2020. "Collaborative Intimacies: How Research Pigs in Danish Organ Transplantation Facilitate Medical Training, Moral Reflection and Social Networking." *Medicine Anthropology Theory* 7 (2): 120–149.

Jensen, Claus Aastrup, Nikolaj Malchow-Møller, Jakob Roland Munch, and Jan Rose Skaksen. 2007. *Udenlandsk arbejdskraft i landbruget: Omfang, udvikling og konsekvenser* [Foreign Labor in Agriculture: Scope, Development and Consequences]. Copenhagen: Rockwool Foundation Research Unit.

Jensen, Henrik. 2016. *Derfra vores verden går: Et essay om fædrelandskærlighed* [From There Our World Goes: An Essay on Patriotism]. Copenhagen: Kristeligt Dagblads Forlag.

Jensen, Michael L., Per T. Sangild, Mikkel Lykke, Mette Schmidt, Mette Boye, Bent B. Jensen, and Thomas Thymann. 2013. "Similar Efficacy of Human Banked Milk and Bovine Colostrum to Decrease Incidence of Necrotizing Enterocolitis in Preterm Piglets." *American Journal of Physiology* 305 (1): R4–R12.

Jensen, Tenna. 2013. "The Nutritional Transformation of Danish Pork 1887–1960." In *The Food Industries of Europe in the Nineteenth and Twentieth Centuries*, edited by Derek J. Oddy and Alain Drouard, 133–147. Farnham, UK: Ashgate.

Jonsen, Albert R. 1998. *The Birth of Bioethics.* Oxford: Oxford University Press.

Jønsson, Heidi Vad. 2018. *Indvandring i velfærdsstaten* [Immigration in the Welfare State]. Aarhus, Denmark: Aarhus Universitetsforlag.

Kærgård, Niels. 2017. "Dansk landbrug i fortid, nutid og fremtid [Danish Agriculture in the Past, Present, and Future]." *Samfundsøkonomen* 4 (December): 4–9.

"Kan man undgå at kalve aflives ved fødslen? [Can Calf Deaths at Birth Be Avoided?]." N.d. *Mejeri.dk.* Accessed April 12, 2021. https://mejeri.dk/dyrevelfaerd/kan-man-undga-at -kalve-aflives-ved-fodslen/.

Karlsen, Marry-Anne. 2018. "The Limits of Egalitarianism: Irregular Migration and the Norwegian Welfare State." In *Egalitarianism in Scandinavia: Historical and Contemporary Perspectives*, edited by Synnove Bendixsen, Mary Bente Bringslid, and Halvard Vike, 223–243. Cham, Switzerland: Palgrave Macmillan.

Kaufman, Sharon R. 2005. *And a Time to Die: How American Hospitals Shape the End of Life.* Chicago: University of Chicago Press.

Keller, Evelyn F. 1992. *Secrets of Life, Secrets of Death: Essays on Language, Gender and Science.* New York: Routledge.

Kermode, Frank. 2000. *The Sense of an Ending: Studies in the Theory of Fiction, with a New Epilogue.* Oxford: Oxford University Press.

Kierkegaard, Søren. [1843] 1983. *Kierkegaard's Writings, VI, Volume 6: Fear and Trembling/Repetition.* Edited by Hong Howard V. and Hong Edna H. Princeton, NJ: Princeton University Press.

Kirchhelle, Claas. 2018. "Pharming Animals: A Global History of Antibiotics in Food Production (1935–2017)." *Palgrave Communications* 4 (96): 1–13.

Kirk, Robert G. W. 2016a. "The Birth of the Laboratory Animal: Biopolitics, Animal Experimentation, and Animal Wellbeing." In *Foucault and Animals*, edited by Matthew Chrulew and Dinesh Joseph Wadiwel, 191–221. Leiden, the Netherlands: Brill.

———. 2016b. "Care in the Cage: Materializing Moral Economies of Animal Care in the Biomedical Sciences, c. 1945–." In *Animal Housing and Human-Animal Relations: Politics, Practices and Infrastructures*, edited by Kristian Bjørkdahl and Tone Druglitrø, 167–184. London: Routledge.

Kirk, Robert G. W., and Edmund Ramsden. 2018. "Working across Species down on the Farm: Howard S. Liddell and the Development of Comparative Psychopathology, c. 1923–1962." *History and Philosophy of the Life Sciences* 40 (24): 1–29.

Kirksey, S. Eben, and Stefan Helmreich. 2010. "The Emergence of Multispecies Ethnography." *Cultural Anthropology* 25 (4): 545–576.

Koch, Lene. 2000. *Tvangssterilisation i Danmark 1929–67* [Forced Sterilization in Denmark 1929–67]. Copenhagen: Gyldendal.

———. 2014. *Racehygiejne i Danmark 1920–1956* [Racial Hygiene in Denmark 1920–1956]. Copenhagen: Informations Forlag.

Koch, Lene, and Mette N. Svendsen. 2015. "Negotiating Moral Value: A Story of Danish Research Monkeys and Their Humans." *Science, Technology and Human Values* 40 (3): 368–388.

———. 2016. "Back to Nature! Rehabilitating Danish Research Monkeys." In *Animal Housing and Human-Animal Relations: Politics, Practices and Infrastructures*, edited by Kristian Bjørkdahl, and Tone Druglitrø, 67–81. London: Routledge.

Kohn, Eduardo. 2007. "How Dogs Dream: Amazonian Natures and the Politics of Transspecies Engagement." *American Ethnologist* 34 (1): 3–24.

Kolstrup, Søren. 2011. "Fra fattiglov til forsorgslov [From Poverty Law to Welfare Law]." In *Dansk Velfærdshistorie, bd. II: Mellem skøn og ret—perioden 1898–1933* [Danish Welfare History, vol. II: Between Discretion and Law—The Period 1898–1933], edited by Jørn Henrik Petersen, Klaus Petersen, and Niels Finn Chistiansen, 149–232. Odense, Denmark: Syddansk Universitetsforlag.

Konrad, Monica. 2005. *Narrating the New Predictive Genetics: Ethics, Ethnography and Science.* Cambridge: Cambridge University Press.

Kristensen, Hans. 2020. *Svinevirke: Historien om det danske grænsehegn og om de vildsvin, som det skulle holde ude* [Pig Activities: The Story of the Danish Border Fence and the Wild Boars That It Was Supposed to Keep out]. Tønder, Denmark: Bogjagt.dk.

Kuan, Teresa, and Lone Grøn. 2017. "Introduction to 'Moral (and Other) Laboratories.'" *Culture, Medicine, and Psychiatry* 41 (2): 185–201.

Kuzmuk, K. N., and Lawrence Schook. 2011. "Pigs as a Model for Biomedical Sciences." In *The Genetics of the Pig.* 2nd ed., 426–444. Wallingford, Oxfordshire, UK: CABI.

Lambek, Michael. 2015. *The Ethical Condition: Essays on Action, Person, and Value.* Chicago: Chicago University Press.

Landecker, Hannah. 2011. "Food as Exposure: Nutritional Epigenetics and the New Metabolism." *BioSocieties* 6 (2): 167–194.

———. 2013. "Postindustrial Metabolism: Fat Knowledge." *Public Culture* 25 (3): 495–522.

Landzelius, Kyra. 2003. "Humanizing the Imposter: Object Relations and Illness Equations in the Neonatal Intensive Care Unit." *Culture, Medicine and Psychiatry* 27 (1): 1–28.

Lapegna, Pablo. 2016. *Soybeans and Power: Genetically Modified Crops, Environmental Politics, and Social Movements in Argentina*. New York: Oxford University Press.

Larsen, Christian A. and Jørgen Goul Andersen. 2009. "How New Economic Ideas Changed the Danish Welfare State: The Case of Neoliberal Ideas and Highly Organized Social Democratic Interests." *Governance* 22(2): 239–261.

Larsen, Jørgen E., Tea T. Bengtsson and Morten Frederiksen. 2015. *The Danish Welfare State: A Sociological Investigation*. Basingstoke: Palgrave Macmillan.

Latimer, Joanna. 2013. "Being Alongside: Rethinking Relations amongst Different Kinds." *Theory, Culture and Society* 30 (7–8): 77–104.

Latimer, Joanna, and Mara Miele. 2013. "Naturecultures? Science, Affect and the Non-Human." *Theory, Culture and Society* 30 (7–8): 5–31.

Latour, Bruno. 1987. *Science in Action*. Cambridge, MA: Harvard University Press.

Latour, Bruno, and Steve Woolgar. 1979. *Laboratory Life: The Construction of Scientific Facts*. Beverly Hills, CA: SAGE Publications.

Law, John, and Annemarie Mol. 2008. "Globalisation in Practice: On the Politics of Boiling Pigswill." *GeoForum* 39 (1): 133–143.

Layne, Linda L. 1996. "'How's the Baby Doing?' Struggling with Narratives of Progress in a Neonatal Intensive Care Unit." *Medical Anthropology Quarterly* 10 (4): 624–656.

Leach, Edmund. 1964. "Anthropological Aspects of Language: Animal Categories and Verbal Abuse." In *New Directions in the Study of Language*, edited by Eric H. Lenneberg, 23–63. Cambridge, MA: MIT Press.

Leonelli, Sabina, and Rachel A. Ankeny. 2012. "Re-Thinking Organisms: The Impact of Databases on Model Organism Biology." *Studies in History and Philosophy of Biological and Biomedical Sciences* 43 (1): 29–36.

Lévinas, Emmanuel. 1974. *Otherwise Than Being, or, Beyond Essence*. Translated by Alphonso Lingis. The Hague, the Netherlands: Martinus Nijhoff.

Lewis, Jamie, Jacki Hughes, and Paul Atkinson. 2014. "Relocation, Realignment and Standardisation: Circuits of Translation in Huntington's Disease." *Social Theory and Health* 12 (4): 396–415.

Li, Yanqi, Sandra M. Juhl, Xuqiang Ye, René L. Shen, Elisabeth Omolabake Iyore, Yiheng Dai, Per T. Sangild, et al. 2017. "A Stepwise, Pilot Study of Bovine Colostrum to Supplement the First Enteral Feeding in Preterm Infants (Precolos): Study Protocol and Initial Results." *Frontiers in Pediatrics* 5 (42): 1–9.

Lien, Marianne E. 2015. *Becoming Salmon: Aquaculture and the Domestication of a Fish*. Oakland: University of California Press.

Lien, Marianne E., Heather A. Swanson, and Gro B. Ween. 2018. "Introduction: Naming the Beast—Exploring the Otherwise." In *Domestication Gone Wild: Politics and Practices of Multispecies Relations*, edited by Heather A. Swanson, Marianne E. Lien, and Gro B. Ween, 1–30. Durham, NC: Duke University Press.

Lock, Margaret M. 2001. The Tempering of Medical Anthropology: Troubling Natural Categories. *Medical Anthropology Quarterly* 15 (4): 478–492.

———. 2002. *Twice Dead: Organ Transplants and the Reinvention of Death*. Berkeley: University of California Press.

Long, Olivia. 2018. "The EU-Turkey Deal: Explained." Choose Love, April 5. https://helprefugees.org/news/eu-turkey-deal-explained/.

Lynch, Michael E. 1988. "Sacrifice and the Transformation of the Animal Body into a Scientific Object: Laboratory Culture and Ritual Practice in the Neurosciences." Social Studies of Science 18 (2): 265–289.

Magnussen, Jon, Karsten Vrangbæk, and Richard B. Saltman. 2009. Nordic Health Care Systems: Recent Reforms and Current Policy Changes. Maidenhead, UK: Open University Press.

Maloney, Philip J. 1997. "Levinas, Substitution, and Transcendental Subjectivity." Man and World 30 (1): 49–64.

Marsland, Rebecca, and Ruth Prince. 2012. "What Is Life Worth? Exploring Biomedical Interventions, Survival, and the Politics of Life." Medical Anthropology Quarterly 26 (4): 453–469.

Martinsen, Dorte Sindbjerg, Gabriel Pons Rotger, and Jessica Sampson Thierry. 2019. "Free Movement of People and Cross-Border Welfare in the European Union: Dynamic Rules, Limited Outcomes." Journal of European Social Policy 29 (1): 84–99.

Mathews, Andrew S. 2011. Instituting Nature: Authority, Expertise, and Power in Mexican Forests. Cambridge, MA: MIT Press.

Mattingly, Cheryl. 2010. The Paradox of Hope: Journeys through a Clinical Borderland. Berkeley: University of California Press.

———. 2014. Moral Laboratories: Family Peril and the Struggle for a Good Life. Berkeley: University of California Press.

Merrild, Camilla Hoffmann. 2018. "Social Differences in Health as a Challenge to the Danish Welfare State." In Egalitarianism in Scandinavia: Historical and Contemporary Perspectives, edited by Synnove Bendixsen, Mary Bente Bringslid, and Halvard Vike, 181–200. Cham, Switzerland: Palgrave Macmillan.

Mesman, Jessica. 2008. Uncertainty in Medical Innovation: Experienced Pioneers in Neonatal Care. London: Palgrave MacMillan.

Miller, E. R., and D. E. Ullrey. 1987. "The Pig as a Model for Human Nutrition." Annual Review of Nutrition 7 (1): 361–382.

Mintz, Sidney W. 1986. Sweetness and Power: The Place of Sugar in Modern History. London: Penguin.

Møhl, Perle. 2020. "On the Border." In The Biometric Border World: Technology, Bodies and Identities on the Move, edited by Karen F. Olwig, Perle Møhl, Kristina Grunenberg, and Anja Simonsen, 71–118. London: Routledge.

Mohr, Sebastian, and Lene Koch. 2016. "Transforming Social Contracts: The Social and Cultural History of IVF in Denmark." Reproductive Biomedicine and Society Online 2 (June): 88–96.

Mol, Annemarie. 2002. The Body Multiple: Ontology in Medical Practice. Durham, NC: Duke University Press.

———. 2008. The Logic of Care: Health and the Problem of Patient Choice. New York: Routledge.

Mol, Annemarie, Ingunn Moser, Jeannette Pols, eds. 2010. Care in Practice: Tinkering in Clinics, Homes and Farms. Bielefeld, Germany: Transcript Verlag.

Morgan, Lynn. 2009. Icons of Life: A Cultural History of Human Embryos. Berkeley: University of California Press.

Müller-Wille, Staffan. 2008. "Leaving Inheritance Behind: Wilhelm Johannsen and the Politics of Mendelism." In A Cultural History of Heredity vol. 4: Heredity in the Century of the

Gene, edited by Staffan Müller-Wille and Hans-Jörg Rheinberger, 7–18. Berlin: Max-Planck-Institute for the History of Science.

Müller-Wille, Staffan, and Hans-Jörg Rheinberger. 2005. Introduction to *A Cultural History of Heredity vol. 3: Nineteenth and Early Twentieth Centuries,* edited by Staffan Müller-Wille and Hans-Jörg Rheinberger, 3–7. Berlin: Max-Planck-Institute for the History of Science.

Munro, Rolland. 2004. "Punctualizing Identity: Time and the Demanding Relation." *Sociology* 38 (2): 293–311.

Murphy, Michelle. 2017. *The Economization of Life.* Durham, NC: Duke University Press.

Navne, Laura E., and Mette N. Svendsen. 2018. "Careography: Staff Experiences of Navigating Decisions in Neonatology in Denmark." *Medical Anthropology* 37 (3): 253–266.

———. 2019. "Life-and-Death Decisions in a Neonatal Intensive Care Unit in Denmark: The Discrete Authority of Origin Stories." *Ethnos* 84 (2): 344–361.

Navne, Laura E., Mette N. Svendsen, and Tine M. Gammeltoft. 2018. "The Attachment Imperative: Parental Experiences of Relation-Making in a Danish Neonatal Intensive Care Unit." *Medical Anthropology Quarterly* 32 (1): 120–137.

Nelson, Nicole C. 2018. *Model Behavior: Animal Experiments, Complexity, and the Genetics of Psychiatric Disorders.* Chicago: University of Chicago Press.

Nepstad, Daniel C., Claudia M. Stickler, and Oriana T. Almeida. 2006. "Globalization of the Amazon Soy and Beef Industries: Opportunities for Conservation." *Conservation Biology* 20 (6): 1595–1603.

Nexø, Sniff A. 2009. "Gode liv, dårlige liv—Problematiseringer og valg i dansk abortpolitik [Good Lives, Bad Lives—Problematizations and Choices in Danish Abortion Policy]." In *Folkesundhed—I et kritisk perspektiv* [Public Health—In a Critical Perspective], edited by Stinne Glasdam, 372–398. Copenhagen: Nyt Nordisk Forlag.

Nicholson, Daniel J. 2018. "Reconceptualizing the Organism: From Complex Machine to Flowing Stream." In *Everything Flows: Towards a Processual Philosophy of Biology,* edited by Daniel J. Nicholson, and John Dupre, 139–166. Oxford: Oxford University Press.

Norup, Michael. 1998. "Limits of Neonatal Treatment: A Survey of Attitudes in the Danish Population." *Journal of Medical Ethics* 24 (3): 200–206.

Observatory of Economic Complexity. N.d. "Denmark." Accessed March 19, 2021. https://oec.world/en/profile/country/dnk.

Olejaz, Maria. 2017. When the Dead Teach. Exploring the Postvital Life of Cadavers in Danish Dissection Labs. *Medical Anthropology Theory* 4(4): 125–149.

Oliver, Kelly. 2007. "Stopping the Anthropological Machine: Agamben with Heidegger and Merleau-Ponty." *PhaenEx* 2 (2): 1–23.

Olwig, Karen F., Perle Møhl, Kristina Grunenberg, and Anja Simonsen. 2020. "Introduction: The Biometric Border World." In *The Biometric Border World: Technology, Bodies and Identities on the Move,* edited by Karen F. Olwig, Perle Møhl, Kristina Grunenberg, and Anja Simonsen, 1–22. London: Routledge.

One Health Global Network. N.d. "What Is One Health?" Accessed March 19, 2021. http://www.onehealthglobal.net/what-is-one-health/.

Parry, Bronwyn. 2004. *Trading the Genome: Investigating the Commodification of Bio-Information.* New York: Columbia University Press.

Pedersen, Hans B. and Møllenberg, Steffen. 2016. *Landbrugsregnskaber i hundrede år 1916–2015* [Financial Records from the Agricultural Field for Hundred Years 1916–2015]. Copenhagen: Statistics Denmark.

Pedersen, Henrik B., Sisse Schlægelberger, and Mona Larsen. 2018. *Svineproduktion under forandring* [Pig Production Undergoing Change]. Copenhagen: Statistics Denmark.

Pedersen, Lene J., Peer Berg, Erik Jørgensen, Marianne Kjær Bonde, Mette S. Herskin, Kristian Møllegaard Knage-Rasmussen, Anne Grete Kongsted, et al. 2010. *Pattegrisedødelighed i DK: Muligheder for reduktion af pattegrisedødeligheden i Danmark* [Piglet Mortality in Denmark: Possibilities for Reduction of Denmark's Pig Mortality]. Aarhus University, Department of Agriculture.

Pedersen, Ove K. 2018. *Reaktionens tid: konkurrencestaten mellem reform og reaktion* [Reaction Time: The State of Competition between Reform and Reaction]. Copenhagen: Informations Forlag.

Perrin, Lauren and Francesca Gauntlett. 2020. "Updated Outbreak Assessment #16. African Swine Fever (ASF) in South East Asia." U.K. Department for Environment, Food, and Rural Affairs.

Petersen, Jørn Henrik, Klaus Petersen, and Niels Finn Christiansen. 2013. "The Danish Social Reform of 1933: Social Rights as a New Paradigm by an Accidental Reform?" In *Multi-Layered Historicity of the Present*, edited by Heidi Haggren, Johanna Rainio-Niemi, and Jussi Vauhkonen, 105–124. Helsinki: Unigrafia.

Petersen, Klaus, and Heidi Vad Jønsson. 2013. "From a 'Social Problem' to a 'Cultural Challenge' to the National Welfare State: Immigration and Integration Debates in Denmark 1970–2011." In *Citizenship and Identity in the Welfare State*, edited by Andrzej Marcin Suszycki and Ireneusz Pawel Karolewski, 165–188. Berlin: Nomos Verlagsgesellschaft.

Petryna, Adriana. 2009. *When Experiments Travel: Clinical Trials and the Global Search for Human Subjects*. Princeton, NJ: Princeton University Press.

Rader, Karen. 2004. *Making Mice: Standardizing Animals for American Biomedical Research, 1900–1955*. Princeton, NJ: Princeton University Press.

Rajan, Kaushik Sunder. 2008. "Biocapital as an Emergent Form of Life: Speculations on the Figure of the Experimental Subject." In *Biosocialities, Genetics and the Social Sciences: Making Biologies and Identities*, edited by Sahra Gibbon and Carlos Novas, 157–187. London: Routledge.

Rapp, Rayna. 1999. *Testing Women, Testing the Fetus: The Social Impact of Amniocentesis in America*. New York: Routledge.

Rasmussen, Stine O., Lena Martin, Mette V. Østergaard, Silvia Rudloff, Yanqi Li, Michael Roggenbuck, Stine B. Bering, et al. 2016. "Bovine Colostrum Improves Neonatal Growth, Digestive Function, and Gut Immunity Relative to Donor Human Milk and Infant Formula in Preterm Pigs." *American Journal of Physiology* 311 (3): G480–G491.

Rees, Tobias. 2018. *After Ethnos*. Durham, NC: Duke University Press.

Regan, Tom. 1983. *A Case for Animal Rights: The Case for Animal Rights Updated with a New Preface*. Berkeley: University of California Press.

Remeur, Cecile. 2013. "Welfare Benefits and Intra-EU Mobility." *Library of the European Parliament*. Accessed April 26, 2021. https://www.europarl.europa.eu/RegData/bibliotheque/briefing/2013/130634/LDM_BRI(2013)130634_REV1_EN.pdf.

Roberts, Elizabeth F. S. 2007. "Extra Embryos: The Ethics of Cryopreservation in Ecuador and Elsewhere." *American Ethnologist* 34 (1): 181–199.

Robertson, Bengt, Tore Curstedt, Jan Johansson, Hans Jörnvall, and Tsutomu Kobayashi. 1990. "Structural and Functional Characterization of Porcine Surfactant Isolated from Liquid-Gel Chromatography." *Basic Research on Lung Surfactant* 25: 237–246.

Roll-Hansen, Nils. 2005. "Sources of Johannsen's Genotype Theory." In *A Cultural History of Heredity vol 3: Nineteenth and Early Twentieth Centuries*, edited by Staffan Müller-Wille and Hans-Jörg Rheinberger, 43–52. Berlin: Max-Planck-Institute for the History of Science.

Rose, Nikolas. 1999. *Powers of Freedom: Reframing Political Thought*. Cambridge: Cambridge University Press.

Russell, Nerissa. 2007. "The Domestication of Anthropology." In *Where the Wild Things Are Now: Domestication Reconsidered*, edited by Rebecca Cassidy, and Molly Mullin, 27–48. Oxford: Berg.

Russell, William M. S., Rex L. Burch, and Charles W. Hume. 1959. *The Principles of Humane Experimental Technique*. London: Methuen.

Rutherford, Kenneth M. D., Emma M. Baxter, Birgitte Ask, Peer Berg, Richard B. D'Eath, Susan Jarvis, Karsten K. Jensen, et al. 2011. *The Ethical and Welfare Implications of Large Litter Size in the Domestic Pig: Challenges and Solutions*. Copenhagen: Danish Centre for Bioethics and Risk Assessment.

Rytter, Mikkel. 2010. "'The Family of Denmark' and 'the Aliens': Kinship Images in Danish Integration Politics." *Ethnos* 75 (3): 301–322.

Sahlins, Marshall. 2011. "What Kinship Is (Part One)." *Journal of the Royal Anthropological Institute* 17 (1): 2–19.

Sandøe, Peter, and Stine B. Christiansen. 2008. *Ethics of Animal Use*. Oxford: Wiley-Blackwell.

Sangild, Per T., Thomas Thymann, Mette Schmidt, Barbara Stoll, Douglas G. Burrin, and Randall K. Buddington. 2014. "Invited Review: The Preterm Pig as a Model in Pediatric Gastroenterology." *Journal of Animal Science* 91 (10): 4713–4729.

Saraiva, Tiago. 2016. *Fascist Pigs: Technoscientific Organisms and the History of Fascism*. Cambridge, MA: MIT Press.

Scarry, Elaine. 1985. *The Body in Pain: The Making and Unmaking of the World*. Oxford: Oxford University Press.

Scheper-Hughes, Nancy. 1992. *Death without Weeping: The Violence of Everyday Life in Brazil*. Berkeley and Los Angeles: University of California Press.

Schinkel, Willem. 2008. "The Moralisation of Citizenship in Dutch Integration Discourse." *Amsterdam Law Forum* 1 (1): 15–26.

———. 2017. *Imagined Societies: A Critique of Immigrant Integration in Western Europe*. Cambridge: Cambridge University Press.

Schneider, David M. 1980. *American Kinship: A Cultural Account*. 2nd ed. Chicago: Chicago University Press.

Schneider, David M. 1984. *A Critique of the Study of Kinship*. Ann Arbor: University of Michigan Press.

Schwennesen, Nete, Mette N. Svendsen, and Lene Koch. 2010. "Beyond Informed Choice: Prenatal Risk Assessment, Decision-Making and Trust." *Clinical Ethics* 5 (4): 207–216.

Sharma, Aradhana, and Akhil Gupta, eds. 2006. "Introduction." In *The Anthropology of the State: A Reader*, 1–41. Malden, MA: Blackwell Publishing.

Sharp, Lesley A. 2014. *The Transplant Imaginary: Mechanical Hearts, Animal Parts, and Moral Thinking*. Berkeley: University of California Press.

———. 2019. *Animal Ethos: The Morality of Human-Animal Encounters in Experimental Lab Science*. Berkeley: University of California Press.

Shaw, Rhonda. 2004. "The Virtues of Cross-Nursing and the 'Yuk Factor.'" *Australian Feminist Studies* 19 (45): 287–299.

Singer, Peter. 1975. *Animal Liberation: A New Ethics for Our Treatment of Animals*. New York: Random House.

Smith, Brian, and Wendy Doniger. 1989. "Sacrifice and Substitution: Ritual Mystification and Mythical Demystification." *Numen* 36 (2): 189–224.

Solberg, Berge. 2018. "From Prenatal Diagnosis to Preterm Infants: A Cultural Guide to Understand Scandinavian Variation." *Pediatrics* 142 (supplement 1): S593–S599.

Solomon, Harris. 2016. *Metabolic Living: Food, Fat, and the Absorption of Illness in India*. Durham, NC: Duke University Press.

Spalletta, Olivia. 2021. "Patrons of the State: Reciprocity, Belonging, and Life with Down Syndrome in Denmark." PhD diss., Brandeis University.

Squier, Susan Merrill. 2004. *Liminal Lives: Imagining the Human at the Frontiers of Biomedicine.* Durham, NC: Duke University Press.

Stasch, Rupert. 2009. *Society of Others: Kinship and Mourning in a West Papuan Place.* Berkeley: University of California Press.

Statistics Denmark. 2014. "Flere børn bliver passet ude [More Children Are Being Cared for Outside of the Home]." *Nyt fra Statistics Denmark* 146 (March 20, 2014): 1–2.

Steincke, Karl K. 1920. *Fremtidens Forsørgelsesvæsen* [The Social Security of the Future]. Copenhagen: J. H. Schultz.

Steward, Corrina. 2007. "From Colonization to 'Environmental Soy': A Case Study of Environmental and Socio-Economic Valuation in the Amazon Soy Frontier." *Agriculture and Human Values* 24 (1): 107–122.

Støjberg, Inger. 2017. Letter from the Minister to the Citizenship Committee, October 10, 2017. Accessed April 20, 2021. https://www.ft.dk/samling/20171/almdel/ifu/spm/6/svar/1432974/1801575/index.htm.

Støy, Ann Cathrine F., Peter M. H. Heegaard, Thomas Thymann, Mette Bjerre, Kerstin Skovgaard, Mette Boye, Barbara Stoll, et al. 2014. "Bovine Colostrum Improves Intestinal Function Following Formula-Induced Gut Inflammation in Preterm Pigs." *Clinical Nutrition* 33 (2): 322–329.

Strathern, Marilyn 1992a. *After Nature: English Kinship in the Late Twentieth Century.* Cambridge: Cambridge University Press.

———. 1992b. *Reproducing the Future: Anthropology, Kinship, and the New Reproductive Technologies.* London: Routledge.

"substitution, n." March 2021. OED Online. Accessed April 8 2021. https://www.oed.com/view/Entry/193085?redirectedFrom=substitution&.

Sullivan, Tory P., William H. Eaglstein, Stephen C. Davis, and Patricia Mertz. 2001. "The Pig as a Model for Human Wound Healing." *Wound Repair and Regeneration* 9 (2): 66–76.

Svendsen, Mette N. 2007. "Between Reproductive and Regenerative Medicine: Practising Embryo Donation and Civil Responsibility in Denmark." *Body and Society* 13 (4): 21–46.

———. 2009. "Kritisk Engageret Videnskab: Erfaringer fra forskning i gen- og forplantningsteknologier [Critically Engaged Science: Experiences from Research in Gene and Reproductive Technologies]." *Tidsskrift for Forskning i Sygdom og Samfund* 6 (10): 37–57.

———. 2011. "Articulating Potentiality: Notes on the Delineation of the Blank Figure in Human Embryonic Stem Cell Research." *Cultural Anthropology* 26 (3): 414–437.

———. 2015. "Selective Reproduction: Social and Temporal Imaginaries for Negotiating the Value of Life in Human and Animal Neonates." *Medical Anthropology Quarterly* 29 (2): 178–195.

———. 2016. "The Spatial Arrangements of Making Research Piglets into Resources." In *Animal Housing and Human-Animal Relations: Politics, Practices and Infrastructures*, edited by Kristian Bjørkdahl, and Tone Druglitrø, 185–198. London: Routledge.

———. 2017. "Pigs in Public Health." *Critical Public Health* 27 (3): 384–390.

———. 2020. "Pig-Human Relations in Neonatology: Knowing and Unknowing in a Multispecies Collaborative." In *Biosocial Worlds: Anthropology and Health Environments beyond Determinism*, edited by Jens Seeberg, Andreas Roepstorff, and Lotte Meinert, 69–90. London: UCL Press.

Svendsen, Mette N., Iben M. Gjødsbøl, Mie S. Dam, and Laura E. Navne. 2017. "Humanity at the Edge: The Moral Laboratory of Feeding Precarious Lives." *Culture, Medicine, and Psychiatry* 41 (2): 202–223.

Svendsen, Mette N., and Lene Koch. 2008. "Unpacking the 'Spare Embryo': Facilitating Stem Cell Research in a Moral Landscape." *Social Studies of Science* 38 (1): 93–110.

———. 2013. "Potentializing the Research Piglet in Experimental Neonatal Research." *Current Anthropology* 54 (supplement 7): 118–128.

Svendsen, Mette N., Laura E. Navne, Iben M. Gjødsbøl, and Mie S. Dam. 2018. "A Life Worth Living: Temporality, Care and Personhood." *American Ethnologist* 45 (1): 20–33.

Swanson, Heather A., Marianne E. Lien, and Gro B. Ween, eds. 2018. *Domestication Gone Wild: Politics and Practices of Multispecies Relations*. Durham, NC: Duke University Press.

Swindle, M. M., A. Makin, A. J. Herron, F. J. Clubb Jr., and K. S. Frazier. 2012. "Swine as Models in Biomedical Research and Toxicology Testing." *Veterinary Pathology* 49 (2): 344–356.

Taylor, Janelle S. 2008. *The Public Life of the Fetal Sonogram: Technology, Consumption, and the Politics of Reproduction*. New Brunswick, NJ: Rutgers University Press.

———. 2011. "The Moral Aesthetics of Simulated Suffering in Standardized Patient Performances." *Culture, Medicine, and Psychiatry* 35: 134–162.

———. 2017. "Engaging with Dementia: Moral Experiments in Art and Friendship." *Culture, Medicine, and Psychiatry* 41: 284–303.

Thompson, Charis. 2005. *Making Parents: The Ontological Choreography of Reproductive Technologies*. Cambridge, MA: MIT Press.

———. 2013. *Good Science: The Ethical Choreography of Stem Cell Research*. Cambridge, MA: MIT Press.

Thompson, Michael. 1979. *Rubbish Theory: The Creation and Destruction of Value*. Oxford: Oxford University Press.

Ticktin, Miriam. 2011. *Casualities of Care: Immigration and the Politics of Humanitarianism in France*. Berkley: University of California Press.

Timmermans, Stefan. 1996. "Saving Lives or Saving Multiple Identities? The Double Dynamic of Resuscitation Scripts." *Social Studies of Science* 26 (4): 767–797.

Tjørnhøj-Thomsen, Tine. 2005. "Close Encounters with Infertility and Procreative Technology." In *Managing Uncertainty: Ethnographic Studies of Illness, Risk and the Struggle for Control*, edited by Vibeke Steffen, Hanne Jessen, and Richard Jenkins, 71–91. Copenhagen: Museum Tusculanum Press.

Trägårdh, Lars. 2002. "Sweden and the EU: Welfare State Nationalism and the Spectre of Europe." In *European Integration and National Identity: The Challenge of the Nordic States*, edited by Lene Hansen and Ole Vaever, 130–181. London: Routledge.

———. 2010. "Rethinking the Nordic Welfare State through a Neo-Hegelian Theory of State and Civil Society." *Journal of Political Ideologies* 15 (3): 227–239.

Tsing, Anna L. 2015. *The Mushroom at the End of the World: On the Possibility of Life in Capitalist Ruins*. Princeton, NJ: Princeton University Press.

Turner, Victor. 1969. *The Ritual Process: Structure and Anti-Structure*. London: Aldine.

U.S. Department of Health and Human Services. N.d. "Pigs." Accessed April 12, 2021. https://ori.hhs.gov/education/products/ncstate/pig.htm.

U.K. Department of Health and Social Security. 1984. *Report of the Committee of Inquiry into Human Fertilisation and Embryology*. London: Her Majesty's Stationery Office.

U.S. President's Commission for the Study of Ethical Problems in Medicine and Biomedical and Behavioral Research. 1982. *Splicing Life: A Report on the Social and Ethical Issues of Genetic Engineering with Human Beings*. Washington: US Government Printing Office.

Vallgårda, Signild. 2003. *Folkesundhed som politik. Danmark og Sverige fra 1930 til i dag* [Public Health as Politics. Denmark and Sweden from 1930 to Today]. Aarhus, Denmark: Aarhus Universitetsforlag.

Van Beneden, Pierre J. 1876. *Animal Parasites and Messmates*. London: Henry S. King and Company.

Van Reekum, Rogier, and Willem Schinkel. 2017. "Drawing Lines, Enacting Migration: Visual Prostheses of Bordering Europe." *Public Culture* 29 (1): 27–51.

Vogel, Ida. 2017. "Genetiske sygdomme (prænatal diagnostik) [Genetic Diseases (Prenatal Diagnosis)]." Den Store Danske. Accessed 9 April 2021. https://denstoredanske.lex.dk /genetiske_sygdomme_(prænatal_diagnostik)

Wahlberg, Ayo. 2008. "Reproductive Medicine and the Concept of 'Quality.'" *Clinical Ethics* 3 (4): 189–193.

———. 2018. *Good Quality: The Routinization of Sperm Banking in China*. Berkeley: University of California Press.

Wahlberg, Ayo, and Tine M. Gammeltoft. 2018. "Introduction: Kinds of Children." In *Selective Reproduction in the 21st Century*, edited by Ayo Wahlberg and Tine M. Gammeltoft, 1–24. Cham, Switzerland: Palgrave Macmillan.

Waldby, Catherine, and Robert Mitchell. 2006. *Tissue Economies: Blood, Organs, and Cell Lines in Late Capitalism*. Durham, NC: Duke University Press.

Weiss, Brad. 2016. *Real Pigs: Shifting Values in the Field of Local Pork*. Durham, NC: Duke University Press.

Weston, Kath. 2018. *Animate Planet: Making Visceral Sense of Living in a High-Tech Ecologically Damaged World*. Durham, NC: Duke University Press.

Willerslev, Rane. 2007. *Soul Hunters: Hunting, Animism, and Personhood among the Siberian Yukaghirs*. Berkeley: University of California Press.

———. 2009. "The Optimal Sacrifice: A Study of Voluntary Death among the Siberian Chukchi." *American Ethnologist* 36 (4): 693–704.

Wilson, Elizabeth A. 2015. *Gut Feminism*. Durham, NC: Duke University Press.

Wilson, Kristin J. 2018. *Others' Milk: The Potential of Exceptional Breastfeeding*. New Brunswick, NJ: Rutgers University Press.

Wolfe, Cary. 2010. *What Is Posthumanism?* Minneapolis: University of Minnesota Press.

Wool, Zoë H. 2015. *After War: The Weight of Life at Walter Reed*. Durham, NC: Duke University Press.

Woolgar, Steve. 1991. "Configuring the User: The Case of Usability Trials." In *A Sociology of Monsters: Essays on Power, Technology, and Domination*, edited by John Law, 57–102. London: Routledge.

Woolgar, Steve, and Javier Lezaun. 2013. "The Wrong Bin Bag: A Turn to Ontology in Science and Technology Studies?" *Social Studies of Science* 43 (3): 321–340.

Yan, Yunxiang. 2016. "Intergenerational Intimacy in and Descending Familism in Rural North China." *American Anthropologist* 118 (2): 244–257.

Yates-Doerr, Emily. 2015. "Does Meat Come from Animals? A Multispecies Approach to Classification and Belonging in Highland Guatemala." *American Ethnologist* 42 (2): 309–323.

Yuval-Davis, Nira. 2011. *The Politics of Belonging: Intersectional Contestations*. London: SAGE Publications.

INDEX

ABOUT THE AUTHOR

METTE N. SVENDSEN is a professor of medical anthropology at the University of Copenhagen. She has headed several research projects, including LifeWorth, which explores the worth of life across species, and she is currently leading the research project MeInWe, which investigates the relationship between person and collectivity in the field of precision medicine.

Available titles in the Medical Anthropology:
Health, Inequality, and Social Justice series:

Printed and bound by CPI Group (UK) Ltd, Croydon, CR0 4YY

09/06/2025

14685741-0002

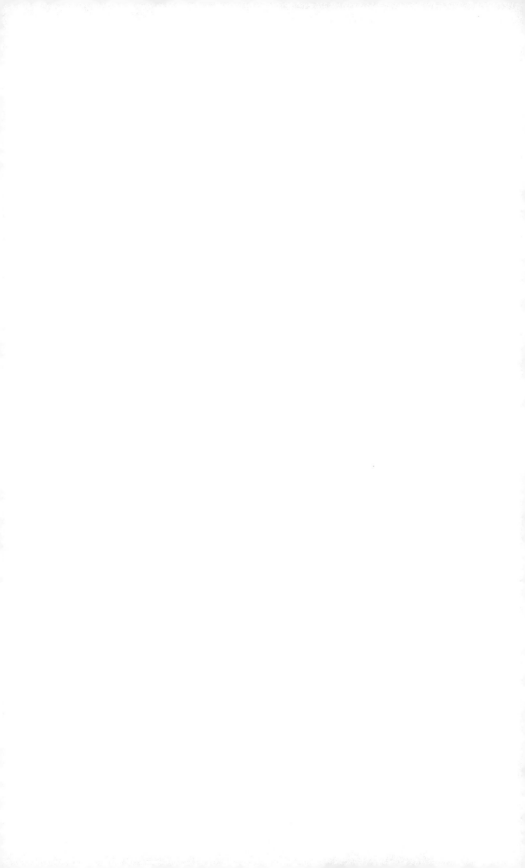